A Guide to Amino Acid and Protein Nutrition

By: **Robert R. Wolfe, Ph.D.**

Professor, Department of Geriatrics

Jane and Edward Warmack Chair in Nutritional Longevity

Director, Center for Translational Research in Aging and Longevity

Donald W. Reynolds Institute on Aging

The University of Arkansas for Medical Sciences

rwolfe2@uams.edu

Published by Book Ripple Publishing

www.BookRipple.com

ISBN: 9781521255308

Table of Contents

4

FOREWORD

I believe that essential amino acids (EAAs) will become the most important nutritional supplements to impact human health and disease in the years to come. EAAs can provide unparalleled benefits in terms of muscle mass and strength. In addition, formulations of supplemental dietary EAAs have a wide range of other physiological benefits. Importantly, there are no adverse effects of EAAs. The benefits of EAAs have been widely documented by peer-reviewed research, ranging from molecular studies identifying the mechanisms of action to clinical trials demonstrating practical outcomes.

My personal interest in the nutritional role of EAAs began indirectly many years before I had even heard of EAAs. I was a 13-year-old freshman at Piedmont High School in California. I was hoping to make the varsity basketball team as a freshman. I had the height (6'5"). I also had the inspiration, having grown up watching the near-by University of California-Berkeley (Cal) team dominate West Coast basketball in the late 1950's., including winning the NCAA championship. My father had put up a basketball hoop in our back yard so I could practice my moves until being dragged in to go to bed. I had one major problem-I was a rail-thin 165 lbs. When practice started in the fall, it became evident quite quickly that the older, stronger players could easily push me around the court. Disappointingly, I was almost immediately relegated to the junior varsity. I vowed to build up my muscles over the next year and not suffer the same fate again my sophomore year.

The problem was that I didn't really know how to build up my muscles. I intuitively understood the role of nutrition, and I was anxious to learn about anything that would unlock the secret to gaining muscle mass and strength. I couldn't find anything helpful, so I just devoted myself to eating as much as I could. I always had a can of a nutritional supplement called "Nutriment" close by so I could force down more calories between meals. I even slugged down a tablespoon of wheat germ oil every day. I wasn't clear on the benefits of wheat germ oil, but I had heard it was good for you and I was willing to try anything that might help. I was searching for any nutritional approach that would promote building muscle. Little did I know that EAAs held the key.

In those days, we didn't know much about the value of weight lifting for sports, but I had the huge advantage of going to a gym that had recently been opened by the now-famous fitness guru Jack LaLanne in the same building in which my father worked. The weight-training helped me to gain strength, but I still didn't gain the muscle mass I was hoping for. While Mr. LaLanne had many convictions regarding nutrition, they were mostly focused on greenish concoctions mixed up in a blender. EAAs were neither *1950's OR 1960's* available nor understood to be the key to working in conjunction with weight lifting to build muscle.

Although I was able to get strong enough to make the varsity as a sophomore, and eventually to have a successful career at Cal and ultimately to be drafted by the Warriors in the NBA, I never weighed more than 190 lbs. I now look back at that time and think about how my basketball career would have benefitted from my current understanding of muscle metabolism and the important role EAAs play in developing muscle mass and strength, particularly when taken in conjunction with weight lifting.

My interest in nutrition and training to improve my own athletic performance took an unexpected turn when I took a class in exercise physiology at Cal. Doctor Jack Wilmore, who at the time was a young professor, but who would eventually become a world-renowned exercise physiologist, taught the course. His tremendous grasp of the subject, coupled with his enthusiasm, inspired me to make a career exploring how to improve physical performance, and ultimately, overall health and quality of life, through optimizing protein and amino acid nutrition.

As I grew older, the focus of my personal interest in EAAs evolved. When my basketball career ended, my athletic interests changed to running marathons competitively. Just as I had found very limited useful formation about nutrition and gaining muscle mass and strength, there was even less written about amino acid and protein nutrition and training for an endurance sport like distance running. As I embarked on my academic career, my interest in both nutrition and training started to grow. I was fortunate to be able to combine these two interests. As a young researcher, I was in a position to start finding out answers for myself. I performed the first series of studies of amino acid and protein metabolism in relation to exercise. These studies made clear that the EAAs, particularly leucine, were a preferred substrate for oxidation during aerobic exercise, and that replacement through nutritional supplementation provided positive results. I extended my early studies of EAA metabolism in exercise to studies relating to fat and carbohydrate metabolism to overall nutrition for endurance exercise. I had the opportunity to study exercise in all types of subjects, from obese individuals who were completely out of shape to world-class cyclists and swimmers in my role as a special consultant to the US Olympic Committee. I also served as a member of the nutrition subcommittee of the International Olympic Committee. Through these personal and professional experiences, I developed a solid understanding of the metabolic response to aerobic exercise at the scientific level. More relevant to this book, I was able to learn how to translate the scientific research to practical implementation in athletes ranging from elite Olympians to the recreational week-end warrior. These experiences led me to develop a program that combines the optimal basic diet and training with judicious use of EAA supplements. I have called the program Essential Amino Acid Solutions for Everyone, or EAASE. The EAASE program has specific applications for power and endurance sports; in addition, as the name implies, there is an EAASE program for virtually all physiological and clinical circumstance.

I recently celebrated my seventieth birthday. Things I never thought of in my younger days are now of concern, especially my diminishing strength and ability to do things that were so easy

8

even just a few years ago, my expanding waistline, and my lower level of energy. Recovery from surgeries has unfortunately also become an issue—ankle and knee surgeries and a hip replacement so far. The EAASE program for healthy aging has been designed to address all of these issues and more. I have been "practicing what I preach" now for a few years, and have found that gradually my clothes have started fitting better, I have more energy, and my blood chemistries have reached the levels of a young, healthy man. Following my hip replacement, my physical therapist commented repeatedly that he had never before had a client who recovered so quickly. These personal observations are not scientifically-valid conclusions; they are just personal anecdotal observations. Nonetheless, they are the kind of benefits that can be expected from a long-term commitment to the EAASE program. That being said, as far as we know, there is no "fountain of youth", and programs that make claims of reversing the process of aging should be regarded with a good deal of skepticism. We can't stop the process of aging entirely, or prevent all major diseases or make Olympic champions out of everybody who trains hard. We can, on the other hand, achieve health goals and maximize physical performance within the context of our inherent capacity.

I have spent the last 45 years immersed in research on human physiology and metabolism. While I have performed studies in Olympic swimmers and cyclists, more importantly, I have dedicated myself to improving recovery from major diseases and injury. As the Chief of Metabolic Research at the Shriners Hospital for Burned Children at Harvard Medical School, I performed research on nutritional and metabolic support following severe injury that translated to guidelines for patient care that are now recommended in both the United States and Europe. After 10 years at Harvard, I moved to a similar position at the University of Texas Medical Branch in which I was able to expand my research to a variety of conditions, including sepsis, traumatic brain injury, cancer, and diabetes. Over the next 25 years, I became increasingly aware of the importance of muscle in recovery from all of those conditions, and in a broader context, the importance of muscle in maintaining health and quality of life throughout the lifespan. Consequently, I moved to the Reynolds Institute on

Aging at the University of Arkansas for Medical Sciences in order to focus my work more directly on health issues related to aging and longevity. I became the Warmack Chair of Geriatrics and Director of the Center for Translational Research in Aging and Longevity. In this position, my main role is to perform research that will directly translate to the betterment of people's lives.

I have published almost 600 peer-reviewed research papers that have been cited by scientists in other articles more than 50,000 times. Most of these studies have been performed in human subjects, and have focused on the development of nutritional and metabolic approaches to support a variety of physiological circumstances. Many of these studies have established the previously underappreciated role of EAAs in a wide variety of metabolic reactions, particularly (but not limited to) those occurring in muscle. In the following pages, I will discuss basic protein nutrition and metabolism, and how the proper use of EAAs can be beneficial for everyone from world-class athletes to overweight adults striving for fitness and health. I will especially focus on the improvement of quality of life that can be achieved by maintaining metabolic and physical function through optimal protein and amino acid nutrition. This will include a discussion of the physiological roles of EAAs and the proper use of EAA supplements to enhance the beneficial effects of dietary protein intake. I fully expect that if you follow the EAASE program described in this book, you will transform your health status and, as a result, improve every aspect of your life.

INTRODUCTION

The Essential Amino Acid Solutions for Everyone (EAASE) is a lifestyle program combining simple nutrition and exercise strategies with judicious use of dietary supplements of EAAs to improve the health and functioning of everyone. Dietary amino acids are the centerpiece of the program because they are the fundamental building blocks of life as we know it. Amino acids are made of nitrogen, carbon, oxygen, hydrogen, and a handful of other elements. Amino acids join together to form protein, the material that forms all of the muscles, tendons, and organs in our bodies. Amino acids are also the main ingredients of most of the biochemical components in our blood and cells. Importantly, essential amino acids (EAAs) are the only macronutrients (i.e., protein, carbohydrates, and fat) that are absolutely required in our diet. In this book, you will learn about the dietary amino acids that keep us alive and how to best use them to improve metabolic function and physical capacity.

I have relied on basic principles of nutrition to develop the EAASE program. A judicious use of supplements is combined with a comprehensive dietary approach to optimize muscle metabolism and provide the building blocks necessary to support the body proteins that keep our bodies going in a variety of circumstances. I also include exercise recommendations that are designed to benefit muscle and overall physical health, and to work in concert with the nutritional component of EAASE. The intent of the program is to augment your normal life pattern without requiring you to completely restructure the way you eat and live. This means that you will not be overwhelmed with a mountain of supplements to face every day. Similarly, my recommendations for exercise will not require you to join a gym and devote hours every day to fitness and training, although I will

11

provide advice for the serious athlete as well as for the more sedentary. The fundamental commitment for most is to incorporate a few changes in the dietary pattern and dietary supplement usage. Engaging in some level of physical activity is encouraged. The plan recommends identifying enjoyable activities that produce the maximal benefits for the muscle and all of the tissues and organs that support life, and how to use dietary EAA supplements to maximize the beneficial effects. While the nutritional tactics alone will provide benefits, the synergy between amino acids and physical exercise is so tremendous that even the most reluctant exerciser will be inspired to engage in some level of physical activity. Combining exercise with the nutritional components of the EAASE program will amplify the benefits to the point where the effects will be noticed within a few weeks.

It is of fundamental importance that the intent of the nutrition and exercise guidelines are clear. The guidelines are designed to become a way of life, not just a crash diet or "detox" to be endured for two or three weeks. Bookstores and the internet are full of quick-fix solutions for health issues, but neither nutrition nor exercise work that way. Although I am confident the effects of EAASE will be evident within a few weeks, the full impact of the program will not be felt for two to three months. While the benefits may take longer than desired to become evident, those benefits will be sustained. In order to more thoroughly convince you of the value of following these simple steps, I will thoroughly describe the physiological basis for the program so that you can understand how EAASE works and why it is a program for life.

I will review the many ways in which amino acids are utilized and relied upon by many components of the human body. The role of dietary protein and amino acids in maintaining function of skeletal muscle will be emphasized. The role of dietary EAAs in liver and brain function will also be discussed. In addition to these basic aspects of physiological function, many other metabolic and physiological processes that are affected by amino acids will be covered, particularly in the context of a variety of circumstances, including athletic training, weight loss, aging, and sickness and injury. Information will be presented that will be relevant to young individuals working out every day to prepare for competition, older but healthy adults trying to slow the inevitable decline in strength and function, or those dealing with specific health issues. Benefits of the EAASE program may be reflected by gaining an edge on a competitor, hitting a golf ball further, or being able to get out of a chair and walk out to get the mail, depending on the individual reasonable goal. Regardless of current physical and health status, I am confident that the EAASE program will help anyone to gain maximum improvements in muscle mass and function and to achieve and maintain a healthy body weight and ideal body composition. EAASE can also assist in the prevention of illness and recovery from trauma such as surgery, or withstanding rigorous treatments such as chemotherapy for cancer. In all cases, improved physical and metabolic function will lead to better physical health and quality of life.

The EAASE program is based entirely on the results of scientific experiments that have yielded clinically tested strategies to improve health, strength, and mental capacity. I have endeavored to explain things in a clear and thorough manner. However, in case I have included unfamiliar words and terms, I have included a glossary of words central to human metabolism in health and disease.

The early chapters of the book contain a basic overview of the role of amino acids in the body. This information will be followed by a discussion of the main bodily functions in skeletal muscle, brain and liver that are impacted by amino acids. The processes by which the body generates energy will be described as a foundation for the EAASE program for weight loss. The ways in which the right nutrients and basic exercises can correct metabolic imbalances and enhance quality of life are amazing. Each chapter will conclude with "Essentials", a bullet-point listing of the key points and important facts on each topic to provide reinforcement of ideas and an easy way to reference information. Finally, the specifics of the EAASE program for a variety of common circumstances will be described.

SECTION 1

Chapter 1. Amino Acids

The term "amino acids" refers to the general chemical class, and consists of more than 300 individual compounds. Only 20 of these amino acids occur in proteins in the body. The amino acids in body protein are referred to as the dietary amino acids because they are also in the proteins that we eat. Amino acids have wide-ranging functions in every aspect of life; they are involved in everything from building muscle and life-supporting tissues to making the chemicals necessary for our brain and vital organs to function. Beyond serving as the building blocks for all-important proteins, amino acids are in and of themselves important signaling factors and intermediaries in many metabolic pathways.

Dietary Proteins - The Source of Dietary Amino Acids

I'm sure you are aware of the importance of protein in the diet, but you may not be as familiar with amino acids. The protein that we eat is composed largely of amino acids – you can think of amino acids as the building blocks of protein. When we eat protein, it is digested in the stomach and intestine and the component amino acids are absorbed into the body. The absorbed amino acids are why we need to eat protein. This process is represented schematically in **Figure 1.1**.

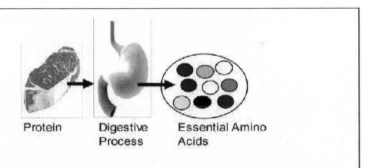

Protein   Digestive   Essential Amino
Process   Acids

Figure 1. 1. There are a variety of protein food sources. In this example, beef is the source of dietary protein. After consumption, the dietary protein is digested into its component amino acids, which are then absorbed into the body. There are nine essential amino acids (represented by the differently shaded circles) that are the key to the metabolic action of amino acids.

Protein Turnover - Why We Need Dietary Amino Acids

There are thousands of different proteins in the body, all with specific functions. Proteins comprise about two-thirds of the mass of the body that is not water. Each protein is distinguished by the unique amount and profile of amino acids. All proteins in the body are in a constant state of turnover. What do I mean by "turnover"? It refers to the fact that all the proteins in the body are in a continuous state of breakdown and synthesis. The balance between the rates of breakdown and synthesis of a protein determines whether you are gaining (anabolism) or losing (catabolism) protein. Most adults are in a steady state in which the overall synthesis of proteins balances the breakdown of proteins.

The breakdown of body proteins provides a steady supply of amino acids to produce new proteins. Even though there is a constant supply of amino acids coming from protein breakdown, we still need to get amino acids from the diet. This is because all of the amino acids that are released in the process of protein breakdown are not available for reincorporation into protein via protein synthesis. Some amino acids released as a consequence of protein breakdown are irreversibly degraded, with the waste products being excreted as CO_2, urea and ammonia. Consequently, we must replace the amino acids that are continuously lost as a consequence of metabolic degradation. Some amino acids (the non-essential amino acids, NEAAs), can be produced from other molecules in the body. However, not all of the amino acids needed to make new proteins can be produced in the body. Amino acids that cannot be produced in the body are called essential amino acids (EAAs). EAAs must be obtained from the diet. In fact, EAAs are the only dietary "macronutrient" that you must eat to survive. If you eat sufficient EAAs, either in the amino acid form or more commonly as a component of dietary protein, the rate of protein synthesis can match or even exceed the rate of protein breakdown. The amount of each EAA that you consume every day is the key to the EAASE program. The relation between dietary amino acids and protein turnover is schematically shown for the case of muscle protein in **Figures 1.2** and **1.3**.

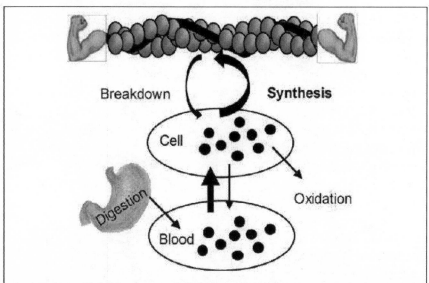

Figure 1.2. All protein in the body is in a constant state of turnover. In this example the muscle protein is represented. Following the consumption of a protein food source, the absorbed amino acid acids travel via the blood to the muscle, where they enter the muscle cells and stimulate the synthesis of new muscle protein to a rate that is greater than the rate of breakdown. Since the rate of synthesis is greater than the rate of breakdown, there is a net gain in muscle protein. This is an *anabolic* state.

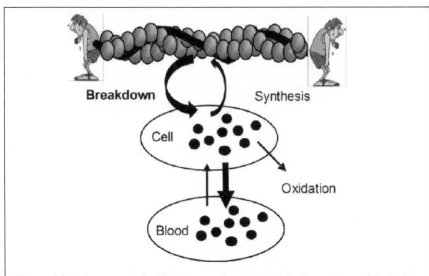

Figure 1.3. Between meals, there is no absorption of dietary amino acids. In this circumstance, there are not enough amino acids available for protein synthesis to match the rate of breakdown, thus a net loss of muscle mass. When the rate of protein breakdown exceeds the rate of synthesis, you are in a *catabolic* state.

It may help to understand the process of protein turnover and the role of dietary amino acids by considering the situation of the body water. More than half of the body is water, and proper functioning of the body depends on maintaining the amount of water constant. However, the body water isn't a static pool- water is constantly lost in urine and through the breath, and if it is hot we regulate our body temperature by sweating. To maintain the body water at a constant level, we must drink water to replace that lost through these various pathways. The rate at which we drink water to replace the amount lost is the turnover rate of water. We consume dietary amino acids, particularly the EAAs, for the same reason (in a general sense) that we drink water- to replace those that are lost due to irreversible metabolism. The consumption of amino acids enables us to maintain a constant amount of protein in the body by stimulating protein synthesis to match the rate of protein breakdown.

We have to eat a significant amount of dietary protein on a daily basis to absorb a sufficient amount of amino acids to maintain the body protein mass. The requirements for dietary amino acids are even greater under a variety of stressful conditions. Many of these conditions will be discussed later in the book. In this chapter, we will review basic information about the amino acids and learn how and why they are perfectly suited for, and in fact "essential", to the dietary goals of people committed to health and their own well-being.

The Chemistry of Amino Acids

There are certain characteristics that define a molecule as an amino acid. The word "amino" refers to the presence of a nitrogen (N) atom in the molecule, and in fact N can be considered the defining characteristic of the amino acids in the body. Very few other compounds in the body contain an N atom. The other defining aspect of an amino acid is that it has a carboxyl group, which is a carbon attached to two oxygen atoms. In addition, each amino acid contains a unique side group that features an element or chemical structure which imparts a specific characteristic or function to that amino acid. The important point is the fact that while all amino acids have the same basic defining structure (an amino and a carboxyl group), the specific characteristic is defined by the side group. Another chemical feature about amino acids that you may have heard about is that they may be in the L or D configuration. The chemical formula of the L- and D-forms of any amino acid is the same, but the physical conformations of the two forms of amino acids differ. The important point to remember is that all dietary amino acids are the L-form, **Figure 1.4**. The chemical structure of amino acids.

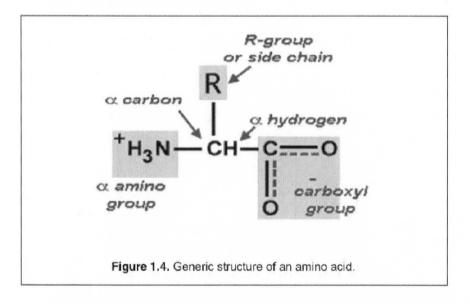

Figure 1.4. Generic structure of an amino acid.

Enough on the chemical structure of amino acids - what really matters are the functions each amino acid plays in the body, and how we can ensure that we eat enough for optimal amino acid and protein nutrition. As I mentioned above, eleven of the amino acids are considered non-essential, meaning that the body has the ability to make or synthesize these amino acids. In theory, this means that you don't need to eat them. However, this overstates the "non-essentiality" of these amino acids. Livestock grow the best when about 20% of the amino acid intake is in the form of NEAAs. Comparable data from humans are not available, but even if that percentage is a significant underestimate for humans, we don't need to worry much about consuming enough of the NEAAs. Most dietary proteins are composed of at least 50-60% NEAAs, so in most circumstances, we consume more than adequate amounts of the NEAAs.

We must obtain the EAAs from food sources or supplements since humans do not have the ability to make them. In contrast to the situation with the NEAAs, there is a recommended dietary allowance (RDA) for each of the EAAs. While the distinction between EAAs and NEAAs is normally clear, in some circumstances certain of the NEAAs become depleted. In this case, the amount of the amino acid (normally considered to be "non-essential") that is made in the body, is insufficient to meet all of the demands for that amino acid. In this circumstance, the amino acid would be considered to be *conditionally essential*, meaning that in certain conditions, such as serious illness, the production of that amino acid in the body is inadequate. This point is particularly relevant to conditions in which the liver function is sub-optimal, since many of the NEAAs are made in the liver.

21

The Dietary Amino Acids

Amino acids affect our health and well-being in multiple ways. You may already be familiar with some of these amino acids since an increasing number are available as nutritional supplements. I have listed all of the dietary amino acids in Appendix I, along with their major functions beyond their contribution to the synthesis of new protein in the body. There is currently a great deal of interest in identifying functional benefits of individual amino acids beyond their role as constituents of proteins. It is important to keep in mind that these functions occur in an environment in which all amino acids are present and maintained in a specific balance and physiological concentration. In other words, no amino acid functions independently and all are required for their principal purpose, which is to serve as precursors for the production of new proteins.

The EAAs include leucine, isoleucine, valine, methionine, phenylalanine, tryptophan, threonine, lysine, and histidine. Histidine was thought to be non-essential for adults since it appeared that only infants could not synthesize it but the results from more extensive studies show that adults also rely upon dietary sources of this amino acid. This circumstance, and the fact that some other amino acids are conditionally essential, explains why different numbers of essential amino acids are sometimes reported.

The NEAAs include cysteine, glycine, glutamine, proline, arginine, tyrosine, alanine, aspartic acid, asparagine, glutamic acid and serine. Regardless of whether an amino acid is an EAA or a NEAA, each amino acid is important as a precursor for protein synthesis. Arginine, tyrosine and glutamine can be conditionally essential in certain physiological circumstances.

Finally, some of the amino acids in the body are involved as intermediates in metabolic processes, but they are not incorporated into body proteins. Examples of non-dietary amino acids are creatine, carnitine, and citrulline. Characteristics of each of the

22

dietary amino acids, as well as the non-dietary amino acids, are presented in Appendix I.

The EAAs and Protein Synthesis

I will focus on the role of EAAs in controlling the rate of protein synthesis because the NEAAs are rarely rate-limiting, since they can be produced in the body. We did an experiment that demonstrated how important the EAAs are in regulating the synthesis of muscle protein. Each subject participated in two trials. In one case, they received a balanced mixture of EAAs (18 g) and NEAAs (22 g) in the profile of beef protein. In the other trial, they received only the 18 g of EAAs. The rate of muscle protein synthesis was stimulated exactly the same amount in each trial. The omission of the NEAAs had no impact on the effectiveness of the EAAs. In contrast, giving just NEAAs has no effect on muscle protein synthesis (**Figure 1.5**).

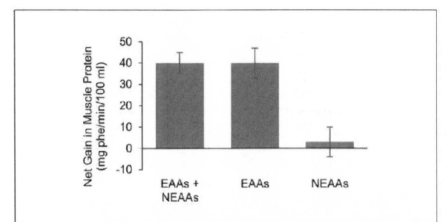

Figure 1.5. Only dietary EAAs are required to stimulate the net gain of muscle protein. A combination of EAAs and NEAAs (18 g EAAS and 22 g NEAAs) in the profile of beef protein were given to subjects in a beverage. Muscle protein synthesis was stimulated to a rate greater than protein breakdown, meaning that there was a net gain in the amount of muscle protein (far left column). The net gain of muscle protein was just as much when only the 18 g EAA component of the mixture was given as when the entire mixture was given (middle column). When the 22 g component of NEAAs was given, there was no gain in net muscle protein. Only the EAAs are needed to stimulate the net gain of muscle protein.

The fundamental importance of EAAs in controlling the rate of protein synthesis, not only of muscle protein but all the proteins in the body, will be a constant theme throughout this book. Furthermore, while EAAs play roles in a wide variety of physiological functions, their role as regulators of protein metabolism is continuous. Discussion of any unique metabolic role of a specific amino acid presupposes that there is an ample supply of all of the other amino acids in blood and tissues, and that the pre-eminent role of all of the amino acids is their contribution to protein synthesis.

Additional Roles of Amino Acids

Every amino acid is a structural component of protein. The principal role of dietary proteins is to provide the amino acids that serve as precursors for the production of new protein to balance the amount that is lost daily through the process of breakdown. Many amino acids play additional roles. For example, arginine plays a role in regulating blood flow and blood pressure as a precursor for the production of nitric oxide, which is the primary chemical responsible for dilating blood vessels, particularly in muscle. Leucine can activate the molecular pathways involved in the initiation of protein synthesis. I have highlighted some of the major ways in which individual amino acids work to maintain a healthy body in Appendix I. However, please don't interpret the information presented in Appendix I as implying that you can expect a specific outcome in response to taking a single amino acid supplement. This would be an oversimplification of amino acid nutrition.

All Functions of Amino Acids Work at the Same Time

When a specific action is attributed to an amino acid, it is in the context of the whole-body chemistry and all of the amino acids working together. The important point to understand about the specific reactions in which particular amino acids may play a pivotal role is that normally all of those reactions are proceeding at the same time in the body. Similar to the way many vitamins function, avoiding a deficiency is important, but taking a dietary supplement that creates an excess does not necessarily create more of an effect. In fact, supplementation of the diet with a single amino acid is more likely to have adverse effects which more than outweigh the specific benefit that is sought. Complications can arise because these functions are not independent of other reactions in the body that are also dependent on amino acids. In other words, most functions that are dependent on amino acids do not occur in a vacuum. Leucine and the other branched chain amino acids (BCAAs) provide an example of how it is possible to cause an unanticipated adverse response when account is not taken of all the potential responses to increasing one individual amino acid.

The BCAAs are leucine, isoleucine, and valine. The name refers to their common chemical structure. Leucine is a key regulator of the rate of protein synthesis. In addition to its role as a precursor to be incorporated into protein, it can activate the molecular processes involved in initiating the process of protein synthesis. For this reason, leucine is often referred to as a nutraceutical, because it can act as a metabolic regulator in addition to serving as a precursor for protein synthesis. Consequently, leucine is a popular dietary supplement.

The consumption of leucine as a dietary supplement is a good example of how all EAAs function together. There are regulatory mechanisms to try to maintain a balance in the availability of all the EAAs, even when an excess of one is consumed. Thus, when leucine is consumed in large amounts as a dietary supplement, the degradation of leucine is activated as the body tries to maintain the normal balance of all EAAs. The metabolic pathway responsible for the degradation of leucine also degrades the other BCAAs (valine and isoleucine) at an increased rate. If only leucine is consumed, all three BCAAs are degraded at an increased rate. The concentrations of both isoleucine and valine will fall below their normal levels. The decrease in the concentrations of valine and isoleucine will limit any effect of the increase in leucine because valine and isoleucine will not be available for the production of new protein. Production of new protein requires adequate availability of all the amino acids in the protein. For this reason, BCAA supplements are more common than leucine alone, even though leucine seems to be the primary nutraceutical of the three. However, even all three BCAAs taken together do not resolve the problem created by an imbalance in availability of EAAs, since there are 6 other EAAs that are not being given. As a result, neither leucine, nor even supplements of all three BCAAs, have a demonstrable beneficial effect on protein synthesis.

The Amino Acids Work like a Team

Let's think about how a football team works, and extend that example to the amino acids. The situation of excess leucine availability could be considered analogous to having all eleven players on offense being quarterbacks. It is great to have a good quarterback to call the plays and either hand the ball off to a running back or pass it. However, he isn't going to have much time to pass the ball if his entire offensive line is composed of quarterbacks as well. Similarly, if the quarterback hands the ball off to another quarterback to run the ball, rather than a running back, the play probably won't succeed. So, although the play can't even get started if the quarterback doesn't do his job, the success of the quarterback is dependent on the coordinated functioning of the entire team. The same is true of leucine as an initiator of protein synthesis- it plays a crucial role, but for protein to be produced, all of the other amino acids must also play their part. Throughout this book, I will repeatedly emphasize the importance of the coordinated functioning of all the amino acids, and the importance of taking a balanced approach to amino acid nutrition as opposed to relying on individual amino acid supplements to address specific issues.

Essentials

- Amino acids are building blocks of proteins as well as signaling factors and intermediaries in many metabolic pathways. Chemically, an amino acid contains an amino group, a carboxyl group, and a unique side group.
- There are twenty dietary amino acids relevant to human biology. Eleven are non-essential (NEAAs), meaning that the body can synthesize them. Nine are essential (EAAs), meaning they must be obtained from the diet.
- A high quality dietary protein contains a ratio of essential to non-essential amino acids of ~55:45, which is similar to the makeup of human muscle. Other proteins contain as much as 70% NEAAs.
- The EAAs include histidine, isoleucine, leucine, lysine, methionine, phenylalanine, threonine, tryptophan, and valine.
- The NEAAs include alanine, aspartic acid, asparagine, arginine, cysteine, glutamic acid, glutamine, glycine, proline, serine, and tyrosine.
- Some non-dietary amino acids serve important functions in the body. These include carnitine, creatine, and citrulline.
- Nutritional supplementation of the diet with an individual amino acid to address a specific issue is likely to have adverse effects on other processes involving amino acids. We should approach optimal amino acid nutrition with a balanced approach that accounts for the interaction of all the amino acids and all of their various metabolic functions.

Chapter 2. Basic Physiology: Skeletal Muscle

Muscle and Physical Performance

When I was younger and trying to get bigger and stronger in order to improve my chances of making the high school basketball team, I didn't think about any physiological role of muscle beyond its importance in strength and physical function. My focus on improving my physical performance by getting bigger and stronger was common in those days and, even today, is the main way in which people think about muscle. This is understandable, since indeed our physical capacity is important throughout our life. In my own case with advancing age, my focus shifted from competition in basketball and then marathon racing to less strenuous activities like golf, but physical performance has remained important to me throughout my life. Since you are reading this book, you too are probably interested in maintaining or improving your physical function at some level. Even so, you may not be consciously thinking much about the importance of maintaining or improving muscle mass and function to your overall health. The first time you are likely to really think about physical function may be when you have trouble doing something that used to be routine, such as walking up a flight of stairs or carrying the groceries in from the car. Or, it could be after surgery, or maybe a prolonged period of missed workouts when you realize how much weaker you feel. Unfortunately, once you have started to lose a significant amount of physical capacity, it is difficult to reverse the decline. It is like closing the barn door after the horse gets out.

The primary purpose of the EAASE program is to help you incorporate optimal amino acid nutrition and exercise into your life before "the horse gets out of the barn". Of course, it is better to start the program late than never, but the optimal time to begin is before you realize how much you need it. This is particularly true with regard to muscle, because muscle plays a key role in many physiological functions in addition to physical function that you may not appreciate.

I can speak from personal experience when I say that most people think of muscle only with regard to physical activity, regardless of their age or health. I can remember telling my 95 year old mother several years ago about a paper I was writing entitled "The underappreciated role of muscle in health and disease" in which I reviewed the central role that muscle plays in the regulation of metabolism in the body, the support of bone health, enabling greater survival in the case of heart failure and cancer and even affording psychological support. I told her about my work with EAAs and how they would help her in her daily life by not only strengthening muscle, but also improving all of the other functions of muscle. She listened very politely, and responded "What do I need muscle for? I am just playing bridge all day. I don't need to be strong for that". My experience with many, many more people since then is that most people only think of physical performance when thinking about the importance of muscle.

Muscle and Whole-Body Protein Metabolism

Muscle has always been recognized for its importance in mobility and physical activity. The role of muscle in maintaining normal protein metabolism through the body is generally underappreciated and only recently becoming fully understood. In the previous chapter, I explained how the entire body is composed of proteins that are in a constant state of turnover, meaning that protein breakdown and synthesis are occurring simultaneously. The term "anabolism" refers to the situation in which the rate of protein synthesis exceeds the rate of protein breakdown, so you are gaining protein in a net sense during an *anabolic state*. The term "catabolism" refers to the reverse situation- the rate of protein breakdown exceeds the rate of synthesis, and you are losing protein in a *catabolic state*.

Anabolism and *catabolism* are most frequently referred to with regard to the status of muscle protein turnover. After all, athletes take illegal *anabolic hormones* to build their muscles. Another reason that the terms *anabolism* and *catabolism* primarily refer to muscle may be something that you haven't thought of, but it is important. Under normal conditions, it is primarily the muscle that routinely goes through periods of both anabolism and catabolism throughout the day, depending on whether you have just eaten a meal (post- prandial) or whether it has been several hours since you have eaten and you are no longer absorbing amino acids (post-absorptive). In contrast, most tissues and organs maintain the balance between synthesis and breakdown throughout the day, even in the absence of absorption of amino acids from the consumption of dietary protein. This is a good thing. Just think of the problems we would have if, for example, you missed a couple of meals and the skin protein became catabolic and you lost a significant amount of skin. Similarly, you wouldn't want to lose any protein from other essential tissues and organs, such as the liver and heart, or kidneys. The essential tissues and organs maintain a balance between protein synthesis and breakdown in the absence of dietary protein consumption because they can draw from the amino acids circulating in the blood. Even in the absence of food intake and continuous uptake of amino acids from blood for protein synthesis in tissues other than muscle, the blood amino acid concentrations remain constant.

Muscle and the Regulation of Plasma Amino Acid Levels

The body is remarkably efficient in maintaining constant concentrations of amino acids in the blood. This is true even in the case of prolonged fasting. In the early 1960s, it was common to place severely obese individuals on supervised starvation. One of the most famous cases involved an individual who weighed more than 700 pounds. He was so heavy that they had to construct a special toilet for him because he crushed the one in his hospital bathroom. This individual was provided only water, minerals and · vitamins for over a year, with the result being a loss of more than 500 pounds. Despite going for over a year without protein (or any other) macronutrient intake, plasma amino acids were maintained at the same level as at the start of the starvation. The essential rates of protein synthesis in organs and tissues were maintained by extracting the necessary amino acid precursors from the blood.

Further proof of the vital importance of maintaining the circulating levels of amino acids comes from data from the IRA hunger strikers. These individuals were protesting the British control of Northern Ireland. They committed themselves to starving themselves to death to draw attention to their cause. They insisted that blood samples be taken from them throughout the starvation so that some medical good may come of their sacrifices. These individuals were not obese, and, in contrast to the obese gentleman referred to above, lasted only about 40 days. The key signal that the end was imminent was when the blood amino acid levels could no longer be maintained. When the amino acid levels dropped below the normal level, the synthesis of essential proteins could no longer be sustained, and they perished.

The skeletal muscle plays a key role in maintaining the plasma amino acids levels in the absence of absorption of dietary amino acids from digested protein. The 700 pound man was able to go for a year without food because, when he started the fast, not only was his fat mass increased, so too was his muscle mass. This is because his diet included large amounts of protein in addition to fat and carbohydrate. Consequently, even with a 500 pound weight loss, he maintained sufficient muscle protein to supply the blood with enough amino acids to support protein synthesis in other tissues and organs. The IRA hunger strikers, on the other hand, were thin to begin with and, by comparison, didn't have much muscle. The point at which they could no longer maintain the necessary plasma concentrations of amino acids corresponded to when their muscle was virtually completely depleted.

You can consider muscle to be the reservoir of amino acids for the rest of the body. The muscle is the only tissue in the body that can afford to lose some of its mass without impairment of health. In the absence of absorption of dietary amino acids, there is a net breakdown of muscle protein to supply amino acids to the blood to balance the amount taken up by the tissues in order to maintain synthesis rates in other tissues and organs. The result is a net loss of skeletal muscle (catabolic state) in the absence of dietary protein intake. When the situation is reversed by consumption of dietary protein, then there is an anabolic state created in muscle whereby dietary amino acids are taken up and sufficient skeletal muscle protein is produced to offset what was lost during the post-absorptive state. An anabolic state thus occurs in muscle after a meal. Meanwhile, there is minimal anabolism in other essential tissues after a meal. There is no need for extra protein synthesis at this time, because those tissues and organs were getting all the amino acid they needed from the blood amino acids (that came from the net breakdown of muscle). The relationship between the absorption (or lack thereof) of amino acids and the breakdown of muscle protein in the post-absorptive state and the net gain in protein in the fed state is illustrated in **Figures 2.1** and **2.2.**

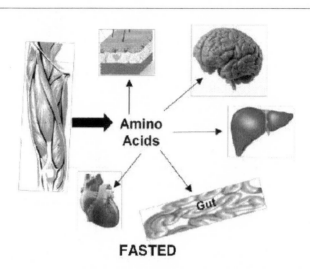

FASTED

Figure 2.1. In the fasted state, there is net breakdown of muscle protein, with the resulting release of amino acids diffusing into the blood for transport to other tissues and organs so that the synthesis of essential proteins can be maintained. Muscle acts as a reservoir of amino acids to keep the blood levels constant even when no protein is being digested.

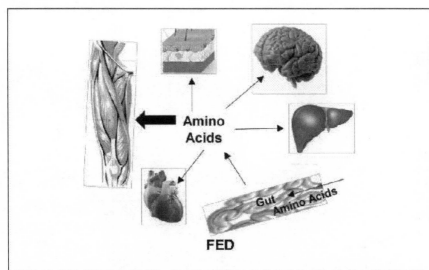

Figure 2.2. In the fed state, muscle takes up the absorbed amino acids and produces new protein to replace what was lost in the fasted state. This figure illustrates how the primary fate of digested amino acids is muscle. This is why the optimal protein and amino acid nutrition focuses on the metabolic needs of muscle.

The schematic representations in Figures 2.1 and 2.2 demonstrate how, under normal conditions, the primary fate of absorbed dietary amino acids is the production of muscle. The fact that the predominant fate of dietary amino acids is "muscle building" explains why the dietary EAAs that are consumed should be in a profile that most effectively stimulates muscle protein synthesis. This point is key to the EAASE program.

In a stressful state, the demand for amino acids is increased. This might be because of increased demands on immune function, wound repair, or other physiological responses unique to a particular situation. In such circumstances, amino acids are taken up from blood at a faster rate than normal to meet the demands of accelerated protein synthesis. To balance this response, muscle protein must break down at a rate that is even faster than normal in the post-absorptive state to maintain constant levels of blood amino acid concentrations. This is illustrated schematically in **Figure 2.3**.

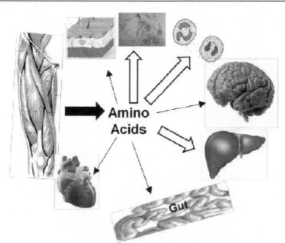

Amino Acids

FASTED + STRESS

Figure 2.3. In the stressed state, there are increased demands for amino acids. This might be for wound healing, immune function, the production of specific proteins in the liver, and other functions. Consequently, the breakdown of muscle protein and release of amino acids into the blood is accelerated. In a catabolic state the stimulation of the breakdown of muscle protein may be so great that it cannot be readily reversed by normal nutrition.

The response of muscle in a catabolic state may be so pronounced that accelerated breakdown persists even after a meal. If this occurs, then the normal effect of amino acids to stimulate the synthesis of new muscle protein to replete that which was lost in the absence of the absorption of amino acids may be diminished. _Anabolic resistance_ exists if the normal ability of EAAs to stimulate the production of new muscle protein is diminished. Anabolic resistance occurs in a wide range of physiological states, many of which will be discussed later in this book. A crucial part of the EAASE program is unique formulations of EAAs to overcome anabolic resistance.

The Role of Muscle in Health and Disease

Maintaining the plasma amino acid levels is the most prominent metabolic duty of muscle, but other metabolic roles are important as well. Under normal conditions, the muscle plays a key role in regulating the blood concentration of glucose as well as the amino acids. Glucose is commonly called the blood sugar. Under normal conditions, the brain relies entirely on glucose from the blood for energy. A drop in blood glucose concentration can cause loss of consciousness and even death. In contrast, an increase in glucose concentration in the blood is responsible for many of the adverse effects of diabetes. All dietary carbohydrates are ultimately converted to glucose (i.e., blood sugar) in order to be metabolized in the body. After you eat carbohydrates, the blood glucose level increases. The magnitude of an increase in concentration is moderated by the release of the hormone insulin, which stimulates the uptake of glucose by various tissues, but most prominently muscle. Once in the muscle cell, the glucose may either be converted to a chemical form of energy or stored as glycogen for later use during exercise when the demand is increased for energy to fuel the contraction of muscle. In diabetes, insulin no longer stimulates the clearance of glucose from the blood. This condition is termed *insulin resistance*.

Muscle is not only important in blunting the magnitude of increases in blood glucose after meals, muscle also helps to prevent decreases in the blood glucose level between meals that could impair brain function. Amino acids released from muscle are not only used for the production of new proteins in other tissues, some of the amino acids released from muscle become precursors for the production of glucose when there is no absorption of dietary carbohydrate. Thus, maintaining the metabolic health of the muscle is crucial for regulation of the blood glucose level in the normal range. This is crucial for the prevention of diabetes as well as the health problems caused by hypoglycemia (low blood glucose level).

The relationship between muscle and bone is not well-recognized even though mechanical force on bone is essential for bone strength and mass. It is difficult to distinguish the role of muscle on bone from other factors, since the amount of dietary protein, insulin growth factor, and testosterone that affect bone also directly affect muscle. We know that weight bearing exercises serve to increase not only muscle strength but also bone strength, and even obesity or a high body weight strengthens bone by providing a direct mechanical force. Prevention of the loss of bone with aging (*osteoporosis*) is highly dependent on the maintenance of adequate muscle mass and function. Regardless of the exact nature of the relationship between muscle and bone, it is clear that strategies to optimize muscle mass, strength and function will provide the same benefits to bone.

Muscle mass is associated with improved health outcomes in a number of serious conditions. Cancer is the most well documented clinical state in which survival is directly linked to the maintenance of muscle mass. Cancer is associated with a rapid loss of muscle mass and strength at a rate faster than would normally occur because of decreased protein intake alone. This is a classic example of the catabolic state. Survival from a variety of cancers is directly related to how well the muscle mass is maintained. How the muscle exerts this effect is not certain, but one aspect seems to be the ability to withstand the rigors of chemotherapy and radiation therapy which is related to the patient's muscle mass and strength.

The all-cause morbidity and mortality due to adverse cardiovascular events (heart attacks, stroke) are also worse in individuals with depleted muscle mass. Interestingly, the *loss* of muscle strength is even more strongly related to mortality than the amount of muscle mass. Survival from other serious diseases, such as chronic obstructive lung disease and heart failure, is also better in individuals with greater muscle mass.

Muscle plays an important role in energy balance and prevention of obesity. The process of continuous synthesis and breakdown of muscle (muscle protein turnover) requires energy. It is possible to calculate the caloric cost of muscle protein turnover. Every 10 kg difference in lean mass translates to a difference in energy expenditure of $\approx$100 kcal/d. This means that a well-muscled man who has 30 kg more muscle mass than an older woman, will expend approximately 300 kcal more energy every day at rest, and even more during exercise. A difference in energy expenditure of 300 kcal per day translates to ~30 pounds of fat mass per year assuming a constant intake in the amount of food energy. The metabolic energy expended to maintain muscle protein turnover is an important reason that a young man can eat more calories per day without gaining weight, as compared to an older woman who would gain weight eating the same amount of food. The magnitude of effect of muscle protein turnover on energy balance, when sustained over a long period of time, illustrates why maintaining a healthy muscle mass is helpful in avoiding obesity.

Muscle Protein Synthesis

Hopefully by now I have convinced you of the wide-ranging importance of muscle. It is a central premise of EAASE that maintenance of a well-functioning muscle mass is central to quality of life and health. The metabolic basis of improving muscle function and mass is the stimulation of muscle protein synthesis. I will give you a brief overview of the process of muscle protein synthesis and how it can be affected by diet, nutritional supplements, and by exercise.

The Importance of Genes

Our genes play an important role in determining the limits on what is possible to achieve through nutrition and exercise. We hear the expression "it's in the genes" all the time. This usually implies that there is nothing that can be done about someone's behaviour or body composition. Indeed, this is true to some extent. Our body build or other characteristics that make us all different individuals is highly influenced by our genes. Nonetheless, all things are not determined entirely by our genes. The heart of the EAASE program is based on the fact that it is possible to improve many aspects of our physical and mental state through optimal nutrition and exercise. On the other hand, it is only reasonable to consider your genes when setting personal goals. Just as you wouldn't expect proper nutrition to increase the height of a grown man by several inches, there is a limit to how much you can expect your muscle mass and function to improve, and this limit is set by your genetic material. On the other hand, genes can be activated and inactivated by nutrition and activity, with significant physiological results. The important point is that although your genetic makeup may limit you at some point, you are probably functioning well below what is possible. Just as we all know that we use only a fraction of our brain power, many of us are using only a fraction of our muscle power.

Muscle proteins are assembled from amino acids using information encoded in our genetic material, deoxyribonucleic acid (DNA). The transcription of messenger RNA (mRNA) from the DNA represents activation (or *transcription*) of the gene. Various factors, including EAAs and exercise, may induce or suppress the activation of certain genes. Changes in the activation of genes are reflected in varying amounts of mRNA in the cell. The extent of activation of various genes is an important determinant of how much of each protein in our body will be produced at any given time.

The amount of available mRNA for a particular protein is a factor determining how much of the protein will be produced, since the physical assembly of a new protein occurs on the mRNA. The mRNA determines the profile and amount of amino acids that are assembled. Transfer RNA (tRNA) is another type of RNA that also plays a key role in protein synthesis. Transfer RNA carries amino acids in the cell to the proper site for protein synthesis. There are specific tRNAs for each individual amino acid that might be incorporated into a protein. When protein synthesis is taking place, enzymes link tRNA molecules to amino acids in the cell in a highly specific manner.

The genetic code is transferred to an amino acid sequence in a protein through the translation process. The amino acids carried by tRNA molecules are positioned sequentially as dictated by the mRNA and linked together. One by one, amino acids are added to the growing chain until a stop signal is received. After the protein has been synthesized completely, it is removed from the cell structure that makes the protein for further processing and ultimately, to perform its function (**Figure 2.4,** muscle protein synthesis diagram). As long as there is sufficient availability of all the amino acid components of a protein as well as the appropriate tRNAs to carry the amino acids to the mRNA for linking together, the translation will continue until completion. From this description, as well as the schematic representation in Figure 2.4, it should be clear that being short of just one amino acid could stop the translation process short of completion. This requirement explains why all of the amino acids must be available.

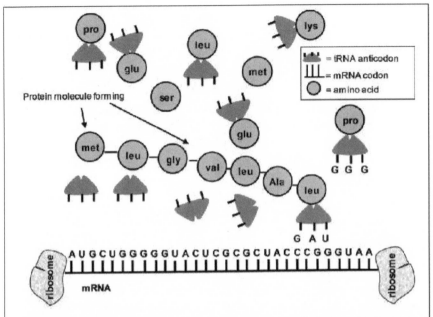

Figure 2.4. Transfer RNA (tRNA) molecules hook up with free amino acids in the cell to enable the mRNA message to be translated. The amino acids are bound together along the mRNA in a specific order unique to the protein that is being synthesized. The mRNA dictates the order of the amino acids. Each amino acid has a specific tRNA.

An easy, conceptual way to think about muscle protein synthesis is to compare it to the construction of a building. The DNA is basically the idea for the design of the building. The mRNA is the written plan or blueprint the builder follows. The translation process is the actual construction of the building. The charged tRNA, meaning tRNA plus its amino acid, represents the delivery of the bricks to the building site, and the actual linking of the amino acids together with chemical bonds according to the profile dictated by the mRNA is "construction", putting the bricks together. The protein is the final product or completed building ready to serve its function.

Rate-Controlling Steps of Protein Synthesis

There are many detailed molecular studies of all the independent steps along these complicated biochemical pathways of muscle protein synthesis, but these don't always predict what will be observed in free living human beings. For example, mRNA may be produced to initiate protein synthesis, but if sufficient amino acids are not available to bind with the appropriate tRNA, the protein cannot be made. Using the analogy of building with bricks, if you add 5 additional bricklayers to the project, the potential rate of completion will be greater, but there must be an adequate number of bricks or the extra bricklayers will have nothing from which to build the building. Alternatively, if there are ample bricks available but not enough bricklayers, progress will be slow. This situation would be similar to the circumstance in which protein synthesis would be slow despite an adequate availability of amino acids because of a limitation in the availability of tRNA. There is a complicated series of reactions necessary to start the process of attaching the amino acids together. These factors are involved in the initiation of protein synthesis and can be lumped together and called *initiation factors*.

Recent publications place great importance on the activation of these initiation factors in the regulation of muscle protein synthesis. A compound called mTOR is the pivot point for activation of the initiation factors. Under normal conditions, the activity of mTOR and all of its related molecules is abundantly available to enable the initiation of protein synthesis. However, in certain situations, such as anabolic resistance, the activity of the initiation factors may become the rate-limiting step in protein synthesis. In any case, the activity of the initiation factors will only translate to increased protein synthesis if there is an adequate supply of amino acids. You can consider the initiation factor activities to be like the starter on a car- you need it to function to get the car started, but without gas in the tank (i.e., amino acids) you won't go far.

Anabolic Stimuli

Muscle Protein Synthesis

Anabolic stimuli promote the growth or synthesis of new muscle. The most potent anabolic stimuli are the EAAs, particularly if provided in the profile that is optimal for the stimulation of muscle protein synthesis. Dietary protein intake also stimulates muscle protein synthesis, but the effect is often not as potent as that of the same amount of EAAs given in the free form. This is because the concentrations of EAAs in the blood rise to a much higher level after consumption of the free amino acids than the same amount of EAAs in intact protein. This largely reflects the different times for absorption. The magnitude of the response of muscle protein synthesis is related to the peak concentrations of the EAAs that are reached.

There are other well-known anabolic factors, and undoubtedly some additional ones that bodybuilders and athletes keep secret. The well-established anabolic factors include exercise (particularly resistance or weight bearing exercise), and anabolic hormones like growth hormone and testosterone. While all of these factors are anabolic in their own right, the effect is modest on their own. The main way in which these anabolic agents work is by amplifying the anabolic response to amino acids, and, in the case of the hormones, the response to exercise. The analogy with the car starter and the initiation factors applies to all anabolic stimuli as well. They all increase the potential for greater muscle protein synthesis, but an ample availability of amino acids is required to be reflected in an increased rate of muscle protein synthesis. This fact is why the long-standing effort to find a drug to prevent muscle loss with aging or serious disease has been unsuccessful to date. Since pharmaceutical companies will only make a large profit on patented drugs, they don't want to link their drug with a nutritional protocol. However, without the appropriate "gas in the tank", most drug therapies are doomed to failure or modest success at best.

The amount of muscle made at any time is the result of the balance between the rates of muscle protein synthesis and breakdown. It is much more difficult to measure protein breakdown in human subjects, so we know much less about its regulation. Most anabolic agents stimulate protein synthesis. However, insulin is an important anabolic hormone that plays a role after each meal, and the primary action of insulin is to inhibit protein breakdown. A large dose of dietary protein or EAAs will suppress protein breakdown in addition to stimulating muscle protein synthesis. Consequently, if evaluating the effect of the intake of dietary protein or EAAs, it is necessary to take account of both the increase in synthesis and the suppression of breakdown.

Factors released in the body in response to illness or surgery can stimulate protein breakdown, thereby inducing a catabolic state. Most notably, the hormone cortisol is known as the stress hormone and increases protein breakdown in a number of clinical circumstances. Chemicals called cytokines are also released in stressful situations and are catabolic. Additional catabolic factors include low-protein diets as well as low-energy diets, and illness. An increased need for amino acids to support immune system function and/or wound healing also stimulates muscle protein breakdown, as shown in Figure 2.3. Myostatin is a protein released within muscle cells that limits muscle protein synthesis. It is unclear if myostatin acts entirely by inhibiting synthesis or stimulating breakdown. Inhibition of myostatin production (basically blocking the catabolic action of this compound) in animals results in a remarkable increase in muscle mass. For this reason, great effort has been invested in developing a drug that inhibits myostatin activity in humans, but there has not yet been such a drug developed that is free of adverse effects.

Essentials

- Muscle is the main reservoir of amino acids in the body.
- Muscle protein fibers are always in a state of breakdown and synthesis or "turnover" which is an important process to get rid of tired, old damaged fibers and replace them with new protein that enable more efficient muscle contraction.
- Muscle serves many important metabolic functions beyond supporting physical movement.
- Muscle plays a crucial role in maintaining constant blood amino acid levels.
- Muscle plays an important role in regulating the blood glucose levels.
- Muscle protein turnover requires energy, and therefore can help maintain a healthy body weight.
- Muscle retains a vitally important store of amino acids needed to sustain immune function and physical strength during illness and traumatic injury.
- Muscle provides mechanical force to strengthen bone.
- Muscle protein synthesis involves DNA, mRNA, tRNA and initiation factors.
- Anabolic factors include essential amino acids, exercise, testosterone, growth hormone and insulin, while catabolic factors include low protein intake, illness and stress.

Chapter 3. Energy Production and Utilization

EAASE is designed to support overall health, physical activity and weight management. The production and utilization of energy is involved in all of these factors. When we think of energy metabolism, we usually think of the balance between calories or food energy consumed and the calories we expend in relation to gaining or losing weight. This concept is entirely correct because ultimately, energy balance is what determines how much weight we gain or lose. In this chapter, I would like to have you think about energy in a slightly different way. We have "energy" that we can feel, such as the desire to be active or feeling attentive and alert, and we have "energy" that is stored in the body, ready to be converted to fuel these activities and brain functions. My goal is to make a connection between the chemical and physiological aspects of "energy" and the "energy" that affects body weight and composition. If I can explain how these things are related and how the body produces and utilizes energy, then you will appreciate my recommendations for EAAs and protein nutrition.

Mental vs Physical Energy

We all desire both physical and mental energy. Physical energy is easy to quantify by applying laws of physics, but mental energy is much more subjective and is influenced by many, many factors. Nonetheless, there is clearly a link between physical and mental energy. I have worked out almost every day of my life. Even so, if I have had a hard day of work and I feel mentally drained, it can be excruciatingly difficult to get a workout started. My mental fatigue seemingly has sapped my physical energy. Once I start the workout, though, it often starts to get easier as I get warmed up. By the end of the workout, I realize that I actually had plenty of physical energy, and that it was my sagging mental energy that had almost convinced me to skip the workout. The most remarkable thing is that once the workout is finished, the revived physical energy translates to my mental energy and I feel invigorated.

My experiences with the interaction between physical and mental energy are shared by almost everyone who exercises regularly. For runners, there is an expression of "getting out the door", which refers to the fact that the first few yards of a run are often the hardest because of low mental energy. Getting past the lack of mental energy is often the hardest part of the run. Another example of the intersection of mental and physical energy comes from so-called interval training. Interval training involves repeating a relatively short, intensive burst of exercise repetitively. For example, it could be running 10 x 400 meters at a fast pace, with some recovery time between each one. This kind of intense workout really tires you out. Nonetheless, there is a well-worn expression that you can always run "one more quarter" (referring to the quarter-mile interval). No matter how exhausted you may feel after running 9 intervals, as long as you know that the 10th is your last, you can always find the energy to run it, usually faster than any of the preceding intervals.

In both of these examples, and many more you can undoubtedly think of from your own experience, mental energy is required to tap into your full physical energy. Figuring out how to tap into your mental energy in a positive way is an important part of the EAASE program.

The importance of mental energy controlling physical energy explains the popularity of so-called "energy drinks". These types of beverages don't really provide you with much, if any, physical energy, but they give you the perception that you have more energy. Of course, perception can turn into reality if it enables you to get started with a workout. There may be a role for "energy drinks" on occasions where staying awake is important, such as during a long, boring car trip. However, the long-lasting mental energy that enables you to complete a physical task comes from within. This is why in the exercise section of the EAASE program, I will introduce you to mental "tricks" I have used over my life to help me get over the inertia and exercise regularly, and to complete workouts once started. In this section, we will focus on the chemical and physiological aspects of energy.

Physical Energy

All of the processes in our body that keep us alive require energy. It is easy to envision the energy requirement of contracting our muscles to perform exercise, but you are probably less aware of the fact that almost all of the biochemical processes in the body require energy. This includes the making of and breakdown of proteins (i.e., protein turnover), the transport of molecules across the membranes into cells, and almost all other reactions. Our "resting energy expenditure" is the energy cost of all of these reactions in what is called the "basal state". Any activity above and beyond lying in bed costs additional energy than what is used in the basal state. A great deal of that additional energy requirement is due to the energy cost of muscle contraction.

Carbohydrates and Fatty Acids: The Fuel for Physical Energy

When you are really fatigued, it is common to say that there is no more gas in the tank. This is a useful comparison to a car needing gas to keep the engine running, to a point. In the case of a car, the motor gets its energy directly from the combustion of the gas that is stored in the tank. In the case of humans, the gas in the tank would be the storage forms of carbohydrate (glycogen) and fat (triglycerides). While the glycogen and triglycerides are indeed the storage form of energy, the body does not get its energy directly from these compounds. Rather, there are several steps involved in the conversion of the energy stored in glycogen and triglycerides into a form of energy that muscle cells and other cells in the body can use.

A more descriptive analogy to the production of energy in the body might be to think of the stored energy sources (triglycerides and glycogen) to be like having gold in a safe deposit box in the bank. It is nice to have wealth in gold, but a retail store is not set up to accept a chunk of gold as payment for, say, a new coat. Rather, you have to find your key to the safe deposit box, unlock the box and take out the gold, take the gold somewhere that will exchange the gold into currency, then go back to the shop and pay for the coat. Just as with the gold in the safe deposit box, several steps are needed to convert the potential energy stored as glycogen and triglycerides into a "currency" that can be used to fuel the thousands of metabolic reactions in your body.

The "key" to getting energy production started in the body is to unlock the stored energy and mobilize it into the blood so it can be transported to the tissues in which the energy is needed. Glycogen and triglycerides, the stored forms of energy, are converted to glucose and fatty acids, respectively which can either be used directly in the liver or muscle, or be released into the blood so they can be delivered to other tissues that need fuel for energy production.

55

Unlike the safe deposit box that has only one key, there are many factors that may unlock the energy stored as glycogen and triglycerides. For example, hormones such as adrenaline and noradrenaline (also known as epinephrine and norepinephrine) are key factors in the "fight or flight" response. When you are in anticipation of, or starting a big physical effort, these chemicals are released and, as a result, both the availability of glucose and free fatty acid are increased so they can be metabolized to produce energy to meet the increased demands of physical activity. Other hormones are also involved in the breakdown of liver glycogen into glucose that can be released into the blood.

ATP: The Energy Currency of the Body

The actual energy "currency" of the body is a chemical called adenosine triphosphate (ATP). ATP is produced from the metabolism of both glycogen and triglycerides. The details of the whole process are a bit complicated and beyond the scope of this book. The important point is that it takes energy to make energy. The actual energy that is used by cells in chemical reactions is energy that is released when the link binding one of the phosphate atoms in ATP is broken. The remaining product is adenosine diphosphate (adenosine with two phosphate atoms, ADP). Think of ATP with three phosphates sitting on the top of a hill. When a phosphate bond is broken, energy is released as the compound falls down the hill, to a lower energy level. That energy is used as it is needed, and then later on when energy is not immediately required, the ADP can be restored to ATP with the input of more energy. In summary, energy production involves the production of new ATP from the ADP and phosphate, and the energy to reform the ATP comes largely from the metabolism of fatty acids or glucose. The more ATP that is broken down, the more energy is required to replace the ATP that was used (**Figure 3.1**).

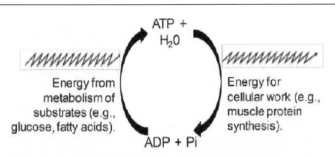

Figure 3.1. ATP can be considered the storage form of energy in the body. The metabolism of carbohydrates, fats, and, to some extent, amino acids converts ADP and phosphate (Pi) into ATP for use when needed. When energy is needed for things such as muscle protein synthesis, as well as muscular contraction, the ATP is broken down to ADP and Pi, with the release of energy. The synthesis of ATP can be considered as a positive energy balance because energy is being gained, and the breakdown of ATP is a negative energy balance, because energy is being lost. If the balance between ATP synthesis and breakdown is positive, you are gaining weight, and if the balance between synthesis and breakdown of ATP favors breakdown (net negative energy balance) you are losing weight. The EAASE program for energy balance focuses on maintaining a high rate of breakdown of ATP to supply the energy for protein synthesis and exercise rather than restriction of the production of ATP by limiting the dietary intake of substrates.

In keeping with the focus of this book, it is important to point out that the metabolism of amino acids can also produce ATP. When EAAs are used for this purpose, they must be replaced by dietary amino acids since EAAs cannot be resynthesized in the body. Compared to glucose and fat, however, only a small proportion of total ATP production is derived from the metabolism of amino acids.

Mitochondria and the Production of ATP

Energy requirements change frequently and quite dramatically throughout the day for most active people. If you go from sitting in a chair to exercising, you need more energy immediately. This means you will need more ATP to enable your muscles to contract. However, there is almost no ATP stored in the body. This means that the metabolism of glucose and fatty acids must be immediately ramped up so that more ATP can be produced. If you are used to exercising, there won't be a problem in producing enough ATP because physically fit people have a lot of *mitochondria* in the muscle tissue. Mitochondria are small organelles in the cell that are the "power plants" of the body. This is where the ATP is generated. ATP is produced in the mitochondria by a series of reactions called the tricarboxylic acid (TCA) cycle, which is commonly called the Krebs cycle after the man who figured out how the cycle works.

Regular exercise increases the demand for energy so, in response, the number of mitochondria increase. Also, mitochondria function more efficiently in active people. On the other hand, if you have a condition such as heart failure that greatly limits your ability to exercise, the maximal capacity of the mitochondria to produce ATP will be quite limited. If your ability to produce ATP is so limited, it can require a great deal of physical effort to walk even just a short distance.

No matter whether you are a highly trained athlete or an older person suffering from heart failure, or somewhere in between, whatever strategy you can use to maximize the number and function of your mitochondria will be beneficial. EAAs can play a key role in this regard.

Amino Acids and Mitochondria

Carnitine and Fatty Acid Oxidation

Carnitine is not included in the list of amino acids that serve as building blocks of proteins in humans but it is an important amino acid. Carnitine is made from the EAAs lysine and methionine. The reason carnitine is important in human nutrition is that it helps transport fatty acids into the mitochondria. Fatty acids are the main fuel for the mitochondria to produce ATP. If your body doesn't have enough carnitine, then the production of ATP from fatty acids will not occur at its maximal capacity. It is very difficult to specifically increase the consumption of the amino acids that make up carnitine-;, lysine and methionine, sufficiently enough to impact the amount of carnitine produced. The supplementation of the diet directly with carnitine is the most effective way to increase its availability. People who are deficient in carnitine will have an increased capacity for physical activity after taking carnitine supplements.

Leucine and Production of New Mitochondria

Earlier, we talked about the EAA leucine and its ability to act as a nutraceutical, meaning that it can regulate chemical reactions in the body beyond acting as a building block for new protein. Leucine has been shown to increase the production of new mitochondria, thereby increasing the number of mitochondria in tissues and increasing the amount of ATP that can be produced. This is one of the reasons that it is important to maintain an adequate amount of leucine in the body.

EAAs and Enzymes

Enzymes are specialized proteins that assist in many chemical reactions. The production of ATP in the mitochondria involves a series of reactions made possible by a number of enzymes. Like all proteins in the body, enzymes are continuously being broken

60

down. When EAAs are consumed, the production of these enzymes is stimulated.

EAAs are thus involved in increasing the number of mitochondria and helping them to work better. Leucine stimulates the production of new mitochondria. Lysine and methionine (or carnitine directly) enable fatty acid metabolism in mitochondria. All of the EAAs are important for producing proteins (enzymes) in the mitochondria that are crucial for the production of ATP.

Energy Balance

More likely than not, you probably found the explanation of energy and mitochondria and ATP a bit tedious and difficult to follow because, in truth, biochemistry can be boring and confusing. You don't have to understand every detail but it's helpful to have a basic conceptual understanding of the dietary implications of the balance between energy intake and ATP production in order to appreciate why parts of the EAASE program are so unique and effective. Like most people, many of you would probably like to do something to change your body weight. Most of us desire to lose excess body fat but some would like to avoid weight gain or others to gain weight in the form of muscle. Paying attention to energy balance is central to maintaining a constant body weight, losing weight while retaining muscle, or gaining muscle mass.

At the start of this section, I referred to the different ways you can think about energy, such as physical energy, mental energy, and energy that is stored in our body. The storage forms of energy make up a significant part of our bodies; fatty acids in the form of triglycerides in adipose tissue, glycogen in liver and muscle, and even amino acids in muscle and other body proteins. Our body weight is very much a function of how much we tap into and use these energy stores compared to how much energy we store away. This may sound like nothing new, "calories in, calories out", but it's a different way to think about and act on that idea.

Most of us are familiar with the traditional concept of energy balance. We think of energy balance in terms of caloric balance. A calorie is the unit of energy we conventionally speak of with regard to energy balance, but it is technically called a *kilo*calorie which is abbreviated kcal. Throughout this chapter I will refer to calories, and abbreviate calories by kcal. If you are in energy balance, then your dietary energy (calorie) intake is the same as your energy (calorie) expenditure. If your calorie intake is greater than calorie expenditure, then you are in a positive calorie balance, meaning you are gaining weight. If you are in a negative energy or calorie balance, then you are losing weight.

We normally regulate energy balance pretty closely. Let's assume you are normal weight and are not too active. In this case, you probably expend about 2,500 kcal/day. If you eat 2,600 kcal per day (just 100 kcal more than expenditure), this will translate to an excess of 36,500 kcal over the year above your energy requirements. Each excess of 3,500 kcal of energy intake corresponds to storage of a pound of fat. In our example, eating just 100 kcal extra per day above expenditure will result in the storage of slightly more than 10 lbs of fat over the year. One hundred kcal does not translate to a large amount of food- for example, one tablespoon of peanut butter more than you actually need. This is why counting calories inevitably is an ineffective approach to weight management. In the first place, it is difficult to know exactly how much energy intake you need for energy balance. In the second place, even if you know your caloric expenditure, it is always difficult to consciously match that exact amount with your dietary intake of calories.

All of the chemical and physical reactions that take place in the body use energy. This includes reactions involved in storing energy and reactions to mobilize energy stores. The energy cost of storing a kilocalorie or using a kilocalorie can be quite different depending upon a number of factors including your body composition or the food source of the calorie. As we discussed above, the energy for reactions in the body comes from the conversion of ATP to ADP and phosphate. Remaking ATP from ADP and phosphate requires the same amount of energy that was released when ATP was converted to ADP and phosphate. Calories from the food we eat provide the potential energy needed to resynthesize the ATP that has been used to fuel the body's metabolism. If we increase the rate of ATP production and utilization (ATP turnover), then we can substantially increase the number of calories we burn.

Two of the most effective ways to increase ATP utilization involve protein: eating more dietary protein and increasing your body's muscle protein. The EAASE program is uniquely designed to activate ATP utilization and to increase the energy you use to build muscle and store away excess calories. What I'm proposing is that you think about energy balance in terms of ATP use rather than calorie intake minus calorie expenditure. If your goal is to maximize fat loss and keep muscle mass and strength, then you need a diet and exercise plan that maximizes ATP turnover.

Amino Acids, Muscle Mass and Energy Balance

The EAASE program for weight management is focused on the role of EAAs in maintaining muscle mass and stimulating muscle protein turnover. There are two aspects of amino acid and protein turnover that are relevant to energy balance: the basal energy requirement of protein turnover, and the increase in energy expenditure after consumption of dietary amino acids and/or protein.

Energy Requirements of Protein Turnover

ATP is required for both protein synthesis and breakdown. More than one-third of the calories you burn while at rest (resting energy expenditure) is used to make enough ATP to fuel muscle protein turnover. The rest of the body protein requires ATP to fuel turnover as well. Enhancing the turnover rate of muscle protein is a good thing because it means that new, stronger proteins are replacing older, possibly damaged proteins. The total amount of energy used to fuel muscle protein turnover is directly related to how much muscle you have and your level of activity.

The actual energy requirement for protein turnover depends on your total muscle mass. To express the concept in more familiar terms, I will convert the energy released from the conversion of ATP to ADP and phosphate to the more familiar units of calories. The conversion of 1 unit of ATP to ADP and phosphate releases approximately 20 kcals. Understanding the energy requirements of muscle protein turnover will make clear why the EAASE program of weight management focuses on maintenance of muscle mass.

Consider the example of the difference in energy expenditure due to muscle protein turnover in a young, healthy woman and an older, somewhat frail woman. The energy released per day as a result of muscle protein synthesis will be approximately 500 kcal per day in the young woman as compared to about 350 kcal per day in an older woman. The difference is mainly due to the greater amount of muscle in the young woman. This means that the young woman even while just sleeping or resting is burning ~6 kcals more every hour than the less muscular woman. This may not seem like a lot, but this difference in energy expenditure goes on continuously, day and night. When extended over the course of the year, the difference in energy expenditure due to muscle protein turnover between the young woman and older woman in this example is more than 50,000 kcal. Every pound of fat that is oxidized releases 3,500 kcal of energy. Consequently, the caloric difference due to different muscle masses corresponds to approximately 14 pounds of stored fat per year. The older woman can only avoid putting on the extra 14 pounds of fat per year by decreasing the caloric intake.

The important point of this discussion is that older people find it harder to keep off body fat, in large part because of reduced muscle mass, not inherent differences in the rates of metabolic reactions or a gluttonous appetite. This is one of the reasons that the EAASE program focuses on the importance of maintaining muscle mass throughout your lifespan.

Energy Expenditure and Dietary Protein and EAA Consumption

After a meal of high quality protein, such as a big steak, you may feel warm. This is in part because energy is required to digest the protein. In addition, the EAAs you have consumed are stimulating muscle protein synthesis, which increases the use of ATP (**Figure 3.2**). The increased utilization of ATP is releasing heat in addition to energy. The more muscle you have, the more energy (and heat) will be released. Obviously, the increase in ATP utilization due to stimulated muscle protein synthesis does not entirely offset the calories you have consumed. Approximately 10%-15% of the calories provided in the protein that you eat are used to process and incorporate the amino acids into protein. In contrast, the storage of fat and carbohydrate is very energy-efficient. The metabolic steps to store excess energy from fat and carbohydrate are much simpler than those for protein.

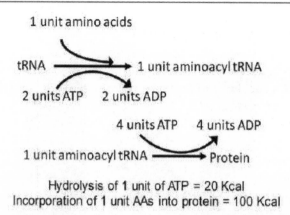

1 unit amino acids

tRNA ⟶ 1 unit aminoacyl tRNA

2 units ATP   2 units ADP

4 units ATP   4 units ADP

1 unit aminoacyl tRNA ⟶ Protein

Hydrolysis of 1 unit of ATP = 20 Kcal
Incorporation of 1 unit AAs into protein = 100 Kcal

Figure 3.2. There are two steps in the production of new protein from amino acids that require energy in the form of the breakdown of ATP to ADP. There is also expenditure of energy resynthesizing ATP from ADP by the oxidation of energy substrates such as fat and carbohydrate. The binding of each amino acid to the corresponding transfer RNA (tRNA) requires energy. The tRNA delivers the amino acid to the mRNA. The actual production of new protein involves binding the amino acids in a specific order dictated by the mRNA. About one-third of your basal energy expenditure is due to the energy cost of protein synthesis. Protein synthesis is the most readily manipulated component of basal energy expenditure, and therefore stimulating protein synthesis is a prime goal of the EAASE program for maintaining energy balance.

Muscle mass is increased by the stimulation of muscle protein synthesis by EAAs. A greater muscle mass in turn favorably impacts energy balance in the basal state as well as following a meal due to the ATP utilization in the process of protein turnover (**Figure 3.3**). Consumption of high quality proteins and EAAs are key components of the EAASE program that make it easier to maintain energy balance because of a greater stimulation of muscle protein synthesis.

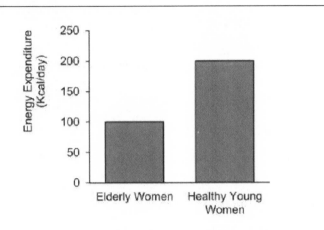

Figure 3.3. The difference in energy expenditure between a young healthy woman and an older woman is significant when extended out over a year. The daily difference in energy expenditure illustrated here translates to the older woman gaining approximately 14 pounds of fat over the course of a year unless she reduces her daily caloric intake to account for her smaller muscle mass.

The increased expenditure of energy due to increased muscle protein synthesis makes it easier to maintain or lose weight while not being obsessed with the amount of calories consumed each day.

The magnitude of increase in energy expenditure due to stimulation of muscle protein synthesis depends in part on the amount of muscle mass. Consider the example above of the younger and older woman. A 50% increase in muscle protein turnover over the course of the day is quite reasonable to expect with activity and a diet containing more EAAs. If muscle protein turnover is increased 50% in the healthy young woman, energy expenditure due to muscle protein turnover will increase to 750 kcal/day, (an increase of 250 kcal). In the case of the older woman, a 50% increase in muscle protein turnover will increase energy expenditure to 525 kcal/day (an increase in 175 kcal/day). While helpful to both the younger and older woman, the younger woman will benefit more from the exercise and EAAs than the older woman.

This is another reason why it is important to start the EAASE program while you are relatively young. By better maintaining your muscle mass with advancing age, it will be easier to maintain energy balance and avoid gaining a significant amount of fat mass.

Essentials

- Physical and mental energy are separate, but closely linked.
- Complex biochemical pathways convert carbohydrate, fat, and protein into chemical energy called adenosine triphosphate (ATP), which is the energy currency of the body.
- Mitochondria are specialized structures within the cell where energy (i.e., ATP) production takes place.
- Amino acid supplementation and exercise increase mitochondrial number and function.
- Protein turnover requires energy in the form of ATP.
- Greater muscle mass uses more ATP for protein turnover, and therefore uses more energy.
- Stimulation of protein turnover by consumption of EAAs offsets ~10-15% of the calories ingested.

Chapter 4. Brain Function

By this point you have probably figured out that muscle is my favorite tissue. Even with my "myocentric" focus (focus on muscle), however, I must admit that, without question, the brain is the most important organ in the body. It is so central to our being and life that it is hard to think of it as just another tissue that requires oxygen and nutrients to keep functioning optimally. As our population ages, many people are becoming aware of the importance of "exercising" the brain and feeding it the proper nutrients or supplements to keep it sharp. Because the brain is so vital to life, it is well protected by a specialized structure that only lets certain molecules pass through into the brain. This protective shield is called the blood brain barrier (BBB) and it is important to the EAASE program because it is selective about the amino acids that it allows to enter the brain. In the brain, amino acids become important chemical messengers that can affect our moods, appetite, energy level, sex drive, and many other behaviors and feelings that affect our lives.

The Blood Brain Barrier

The brain protects itself from things in the blood that may injure the brain by allowing beneficial substances to cross the BBB while preventing entry of potentially harmful ones. In the rest of the body, substances can move fairly easily across the barrier between the blood and cells. We tend to think of movement across the barrier between blood and cells in terms of tissues taking up things from the blood, but it works in the opposite direction as well. For example, amino acids can move in both directions across the barrier between the blood and muscle cells, depending on whether you have just eaten (when muscle cells are taking up amino acids) or between meals (when amino acids are moving from the muscle cells to the blood). In some cases, the movement of nutrients between blood and cells occurs by simple diffusion through spaces in the blood vessels delivering blood to tissues and organs. In these cases, the size of the molecule and the concentrations on each side of the barrier are the primary factors that determine how much movement occurs. Amino acids, however, use "active transport" to enhance the movement between the blood and tissues. Active transport involves special molecules that serve to carry substance into cells against a concentration gradient.

The spaces in the barrier between blood and the cells in the brain are very small. This enables the brain to be very selective about what gets in from the blood. Vital substances like oxygen easily diffuse into and out of the brain, but large molecules do not pass through the BBB easily. Importantly, there are transporters so that glucose (the preferred fuel source for the brain) and amino acids that serve as important chemical messengers in the brain can pass through the BBB. We will see later how the process of transport can influence brain function.

Neurotransmitters

One of the most important ways in which brain cells communicate with each other is by neurotransmitters, which are chemicals that allow cells in the brain to send messages from one cell to another (**Figure 4.1**). Neurotransmitters transmit information through nerve cells which are called neurons. In its most simple form, a neuron has two ends (multiple branches can occur in more complex pathways): an axon and a dendrite. A neuron communicates with other neurons by sending neurotransmitters from its axon to a dendrite of another neuron. The space between the axon and the dendrite is called a synapse which the neurotransmitter must cross. Neurotransmitters are released when an appropriate electrical charge is sent down the axon. Once released, they bind to the receptors on the dendrite of another neuron. When enough neurotransmitters are bound to the receptors, a signal is sent down that neuron and the message continues on. However, if there is not enough neurotransmitter to trigger the receptor, then the message stops. A good analogy is electricity going through a wire in which case turning up the voltage causes more electricity to go through the wire. Neurotransmitters act like electricity in that given enough "juice", functions are turned on and operate smoothly. If the voltage is not sufficient, then the signal will not be transmitted. Once the message is sent, the released neurotransmitters are broken down and the chemical components can be recycled or oxidized.

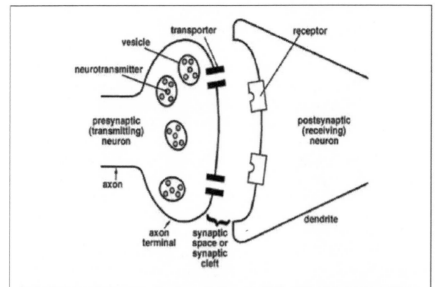

Figure 4.1. Schematic drawing of the junction between nerves where neurotransmitters transmit signals. Neurotransmitters that are released into the space between neurons can bind to specific receptors to transmit the signal. Excess neurotransmitter can be reabsorbed into the presynaptic neuron through the action of transporters. This process ensures that the signal is terminated when appropriate.

Types of Neurotransmitters

Most neurotransmitters are classified as one of two types – inhibitory or excitatory. Inhibitory neurotransmitters slow down the flow of information by reducing the activity of neurons while excitatory neurotransmitters generally increase the flow of information. It is the balance between the inhibitory and excitatory neurotransmitters that is important in proper brain signalling for smooth and coordinated brain and bodily functions. There are over 100 types of neurotransmitters but only ten are responsible for the vast majority of the workload in the human brain. Some amino acids act directly as neurotransmitters while others serve as precursors or "building blocks" of molecules that act as neurotransmitters.

74

The transport system that carries amino acids across the BBB described above can serve to strongly influence neurotransmitter activity, and thus brain function. Some transporters carry multiple amino acids across the BBB, and a change in the balance of amino acids in the blood can affect which amino acids are transported. You may have read about tryptophan in the Thanksgiving turkey being the culprit behind the post-dinner stupor and lethargy experienced by some after the celebration feast. Tryptophan is a large, neutral amino acid that is converted to a neurotransmitter called serotonin in the brain. Serotonin helps us feel calm and relaxed and is very important in sleep behavior such as triggering when we feel sleepy and shortening the time it takes to fall asleep. The idea proposed is that turkey is rich in tryptophan such that blood levels of this amino acid increase relative to other amino acids with similar chemical structures. There is only one type of transporter at the BBB for all of the large, neutral amino acids, which include all the BCAAs and phenylalanine in addition to tryptophan, to gain access to the brain. The amino acid present in greatest concentration will be taken up in the greatest amount. While the "Turkey hypothesis" is somewhat flawed because turkey is a high quality protein that also provides a fair amount of phenylalanine and the branched-chain amino acids, it is true that tryptophan supplements can increase serotonin production in the brain. However, an increase in tryptophan can inhibit the uptake of other large neutral amino acids, including phenylalanine and tyrosine, which are the precursors of dopamine, the excitatory neurotransmitter that counters the action of tryptophan. Thus, a change in the availability of one neurotransmitter precursor can directly impact the transport of other amino acid neurotransmitter precursors into the brain.

This interaction of precursors of key neurotransmitters on transport across the blood brain barrier is a perfect example of the interrelated nature of all actions of EAAs, and the importance of maintaining an appropriate balance of EAAs in the blood.

There are many examples of amino acids working in balance for normal neurotransmitter function. Gamma-Amino Butyric Acid (GABA) and glutamate are amino acids that act as neurotransmitters in the central nervous system. GABA inhibits neuronal transmissions in the brain, thereby calming nervous activity and reducing anxiety. In contrast, the amino acid glutamate acts as an excitatory neurotransmitter and when bound to adjacent cells encourages them to "fire" and send a nerve impulse. The interaction between glutamate and GABA is further shown by the fact that glutamate is a necessary building block for GABA formation. Further, glutamate can be formed from the amino acid glutamine, so the proper balance of neurotransmitters involves a complex interaction of three different amino acids.

A detailed discussion of all the relationships between amino acid precursors and neurotransmitter synthesis, as well as the amino acids that can serve as neurotransmitters themselves, is beyond the scope of this book. The main point of the examples described above of tryptophan and the other amino acids is to underscore the importance in maintaining the appropriate balance of all EAAs in the blood when designing a nutritional program. An imbalance in the plasma amino acids may cause unanticipated and unwanted responses in body functions.

Essentials

- The blood brain barrier (BBB) protects the brain from foreign substances in the blood that may injure the brain.
- The brain has specific transporters to allow entry for glucose (its preferred fuel source) and for amino acids that serve as important chemical messengers in the brain.
- Neurotransmitters are chemical messengers that allow brain cells (neurons) to send messages from one cell to another.
- Neurotransmitters are classified as one of two types – inhibitory or excitatory. Inhibitory transmitters slow down flow of information while excitatory neurotransmitters increase the flow of information.
- Some amino acids act directly as neurotransmitters and others serve as precursors or "building blocks" of molecules that act as neurotransmitters.
- Maintaining a normal balance of all amino acids in blood is important for a balance in neurotransmitter synthesis to be maintained.

Chapter 5. Liver Function

Metabolic Duties of the Liver

The liver is the largest organ in the body and has an impressive list of duties. Its most important job is the detoxification and purification of blood. This includes the metabolism of alcohol. This is the reason that the liver is the main metabolic target of alcohol, and the reason that too much alcohol consumption damages the liver.

The liver also helps in processing and metabolizing the food we eat. There are three major components of food that provide calories: carbohydrate, fat and protein. Alcohol can also provide a substantial amount of energy for some individuals. All of these nutrients go through the "central processing plant" of the liver to be broken down, converted, stored, or repackaged for delivery to other tissues and organs, depending upon the current needs of the body. The liver also produces and excretes bile, which is secreted into the intestine after you eat a meal and mixes with ingested fat to promote absorption of fats.

The regulation of the blood glucose level is a primary responsibility of the liver. Consumed carbohydrates are digested down to their simplest form (mainly glucose). The liver takes up the absorbed glucose and converts it to glycogen (basically a compact package of connected glucose molecules) for storage. The storage of glycogen in the liver dampens the increase in blood glucose concentration that would otherwise occur after eating carbohydrate. When glucose is no longer being absorbed, the liver releases the stored glycogen into the blood as glucose to keep the blood concentration constant. When the stored glycogen is used up, the liver makes new glucose, mostly from amino acids released from the muscle. In a variety of clinical states, most prominently diabetes, the liver fails to do its job of regulating the blood glucose level.

Fatty Liver

The liver can clear fatty acids from the blood and store them as triglycerides, which is the storage form of fat. Normally only a small amount of triglycerides are stored in the liver. A healthy liver repackages the triglycerides into another type of fat (very low density lipoproteins, VLDL) and secretes it back into the blood to be delivered to fat cells for storage. An increased storage of fat in the liver occurs in situations of impaired liver health, such as in individuals who consume large amounts of alcohol or who are obese. Even just the process of normal aging is associated with increased liver fat. Fat in the liver is a sign of metabolic dysfunction.

The problem is that there are often no symptoms in the early stages of fatty liver. Sometimes, a routine check-up will reveal elevated liver enzymes in the blood which is a general indication that the liver isn't working up to its ability. But you can have fatty liver with perfectly normal liver enzymes. Symptoms that may appear as the condition progresses include fatigue or vague abdominal discomfort. If the liver is enlarged, you may feel pressure in or near its location or your doctor may be able to detect a problem during a physical exam. If your liver becomes inflamed, this condition leads to poor appetite, weight loss, and abdominal pain. Compromised liver function can result in physical weakness and mental confusion, and ultimately hepatitis and scarring of liver tissue. While liver cells can regenerate to some extent, repetitive damage usually ends in liver failure.

Fatty liver leads to metabolic abnormalities, including diabetes, and can progress to more serious liver diseases, including cirrhosis. Fatty liver is difficult to treat with traditional medicine. The most commonly prescribed medicine is fenofibrate, which is effective but results in adverse side effects in more than 10% of people who take it, and much more in older individuals. Regular consumption of an EAA supplement is an effective treatment for fatty liver. A clinical trial in older individuals found that EAAs were equally as effective as fenofibrate (**Figure 5.1**), and there were no adverse responses to the EAAs. Other nutritional factors, including nicotinamide and caffeine, can work in concert with EAAs to reduce liver fat even more than when EAAs are given alone.

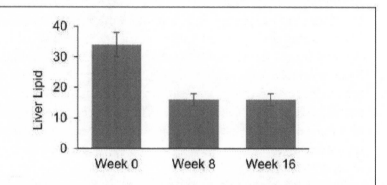

Figure 5.1. Liver fat is elevated above the normal level in older individuals. In a study in which older individuals were given EAA supplements twice per day for 16 weeks, liver fat was reduced to half the value before the supplementation began. The reduction in the liver fat after 8 and 16 weeks of nutritional supplementation was due to an increased transport of fat from the liver to adipose tissue for storage there. The reduction in liver fat as a result of EAA supplementation was as great as in another group who received pharmacological therapy for the liver fat.

The Liver and Amino Acid Metabolism

The liver plays an important role in amino acid metabolism. Amino acids from protein digestion get sorted and transformed to different (non-essential) amino acids in the liver, depending on the need. The liver helps to maintain a proper balance of amino acid concentrations in the blood by producing NEAAs that might be in low supply. The liver also prevents large increases in amino acid concentrations in the blood that might occur otherwise, particularly after a protein meal. When the blood amino acid concentrations increase above the normal levels, they are taken up and metabolized by the liver. The end products are ammonia and urea, which are subsequently excreted in the urine. The production of urea and ammonia from the metabolism of excess NEAAs is one reason why it is beneficial to supplement your basic diet with only EAAs. The NEAAs are more likely to be broken down and produce ammonia than the EAAs, which are taken up by muscle and directed toward muscle growth and maintenance of other body proteins.

So, we see that not only is the muscle involved in maintaining relatively constant levels of amino acids in the blood, so too is the liver. I think it is safe to say that such redundancies in responsibilities reflect the importance of the process to successfully regulate blood amino acid levels. It is for this reason that all dietary recommendations of the EAASE program are within the context of a balanced approach to EAA and protein nutrition.

The Liver and Blood Proteins

Like all other tissues and organs, the liver produces proteins that enable it to carry out its function. In particular, there are many liver proteins that play key roles in mediating the metabolic reactions described above. In addition, the liver produces a number of proteins, including albumin and fibrinogen that it secretes into the plasma. Albumin and fibrinogen circulate in the blood and play important physiological roles in the body.

Albumin serves to regulate blood volume and may also be a means of transporting nutrients and hormones that don't dissolve readily in the blood, including fatty acids and certain amino acids. Maintaining the concentration of albumin in the blood at the appropriate level is so important that a drop in albumin concentration is taken to be the best single indicator of undernutrition. Fibrinogen is an important component of the blood clotting process. Fibrinogen synthesis is impaired in liver disease, and for this reason, liver disease is characterized by slow blood clotting, bruising and often excessive bleeding from the intestine.

Clearly, it is important to have a healthy liver. The wide variety of liver support supplements and liver detox programs available suggests that many of us appreciate the importance of this organ and would like to take measures to keep it functioning optimally. EAAs help the liver by minimizing the burden of ammonia and urea production and promoting the synthesis of many key proteins, as well as reducing the amount of fat in the liver.

Essentials

- Functions of the liver include the metabolism of nutrients and the detoxification and purification of blood.
- The liver is the organ primarily responsible for metabolizing alcohol and drugs and detoxifying noxious chemicals in the body.
- The liver is the place where amino acids from protein digestion get sorted and transformed in order to maintain adequate availability of all NEAAs.
- Alcohol consumption and obesity promote "fatty liver". Fat accumulation in the liver can lead to hepatitis and scarring of the liver tissue.
- EAAs promote albumin and fibrinogen synthesis, two very important blood proteins.

SECTION 2. AMINO ACID AND PROTEIN NUTRITION

Chapter 6. The Dietary Guidelines

What is a "Healthy" Diet?

Most people want to "eat healthy". But how do you know what "eating healthy" really is? We are inundated with advertisements on TV and the internet advocating an incredible range of food and supplements that are all purported to impart some health benefit. A good starting point is to look at what the government-appointed experts tell us. Let's just focus on protein- the only dietary component you have to eat to survive.

The National Academy of Sciences Dietary Reference Intakes (DRIs) is widely accepted by those in the know as the most authoritative reference source to define nutritional requirements. The DRIs are the basis for the more commonly recognized recommendations from the USDA, known as the Dietary Guidelines for Americans, and translated for the public as *My Plate*. The DRIs define the Recommended Dietary Allowance (RDA) for a wide range of micronutrients (vitamins and minerals), and also for protein and carbohydrate (but not for fat). In addition, the DRIs express the recommended dietary intakes of protein, carbohydrate and fat in terms of a percentage of total caloric intake. The Dietary Guidelines for Americans uses the RDAs as starting points to develop nutritional recommendations in the form of healthy eating patterns.

The Recommended Dietary Allowance (RDA)

The RDA for protein is 0.80g of protein/kg body weight/day. For a 175 pound person, this translates to about 65 g of protein per day. In more familiar terms, this would be 2.2 oz of protein per day. An average American diet consists of 4-5 oz of protein per day, or about twice the RDA. This may seem like a very small amount of protein, since you might be eating a 12 oz steak at a restaurant tonight. However, it is important to distinguish the intake of pure protein, which is what the dietary guidelines express, as opposed to protein food sources. Even a high quality protein food source like meat is not pure protein. For example, there are approximately 7 g of protein in 1 ounce of meat, meaning that a 175 pound person can satisfy the RDA for protein for the day by eating a nine ounce steak. However, there are many sources of protein in the diet, some of which you may not even recognize as protein food sources. Many of these other protein food sources have less protein per gram than steak. If you add up all protein food sources you eat in the day, including perhaps eggs, yogurt, or cereal with milk for breakfast, some ice cream or pudding for dessert after lunch, and a dinner with fish, chicken or meat, you are probably eating at least twice the RDA for protein. Add to the obvious protein food sources the amount of protein in foods like wheat, peas, potatoes, soy, etc., you are probably eating quite a bit more than the RDA. For an average size person, this amount equates to ~20% of total caloric intake.

Does eating more protein than provided for by the RDA lead to health issues like obesity and diabetes? This is a perspective that is often suggested by doctors and health professionals. Who hasn't heard the admonition to quit eating red meat? However, you must remember that the RDA is defined to be the *minimum* amount that should be eaten to maintain body protein. The RDA is the lowest dietary protein intake at which the rates of protein synthesis and breakdown are theoretically matched over the entire day.

Dietary Protein Intake as a Percent of Total Calories

In addition to the RDA, the DRIs also recommend an amount of dietary intake of protein in the context of a complete diet. Since all of the food we eat is in the form of three macronutrients, carbohydrate, fat, and protein (four if you include alcohol), the DRIs committee accounted for the fact that the amount of each macronutrient eaten will influence the amount of the other macronutrients in the diet. For example, if you eat a high protein diet, at the same time, you decrease the amount of fat and/or carbohydrate that you eat. Recommended ranges of calorie intake for each macronutrient were set to account for this interrelationship. The DRIs recommend that dietary protein constitutes between 10-35% of dietary caloric intake. They also state that there is no evidence of harmful effects for intakes above this level. For the average sized, non-active person, the RDA for protein provides about 10% of the caloric intake in a day, the lower limit of the range for protein. A diet providing three and one-half times more protein than that is still within the recommendations of the DRIs.

A recommendation of dietary protein intake with a range of 3.5 times (or more) can hardly be considered a useful guideline. Consider if a fitness trainer told you that you could work out for either an hour a day or three and a half hours a day and that either amount is fine and within the recommendations. Obviously, you benefit more with more exercise (excluding risk of injury). In the same manner, you should expect and will experience a different response to a diet providing more protein than the minimum amount indicated by the guidelines. Consequently, we have to accept that the experts have let us down, and that they really don't know how much protein a "healthy" diet should contain. We need to figure this out for ourselves by examining all the recent studies on the topic that are targeted to define the *optimal* amount of protein intake as opposed to the *minimal* amount. This topic will be discussed in depth in the next chapter.

Since EAAs cannot be produced in the body, they must be obtained from the food we eat. Unfortunately, there have been very few studies to define the RDA for each individual EAA, and those studies that have attempted to do so are deeply flawed. As a result, the RDAs for the EAAs are very low, so low that even a diet that would be considered deficient in protein (in terms of the RDA for protein intake) will still be able to satisfy the RDAs for the EAAs. To make matters worse, there are also questions as to whether or not the best profile of the requirements for EAAs was used to establish the recommendations. The "profile" refers to the amount of each individual amino acid in relation to the amount of the other amino acids that are available. I have repeatedly referred to the importance of the balance of amino acids and how excesses or deficiencies of one can influence the others. The starting point for determining the RDAs for EAAs was to measure the amino acids in mother's milk. It is a reasonable guess that the amount of each EAA in mother's milk would be best for growth and development. However, since humans stop growing (vertically, anyway) in adulthood, it is not clear that the same profile that was best for an infant is still the best pattern of intake for adults. Also, certain health conditions and stages of life can place more demands on specific EAAs and influence the requirements. The profile of EAA requirements are shown in **Figure 6.1**. Later in the book when I go into the specifics of the EAASE program I will discuss how various circumstances affect the optimal profile of EAAs, but in all cases the starting point is the profile of EAAs in muscle protein.

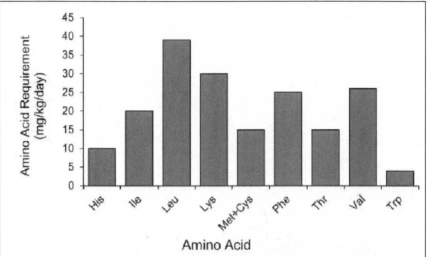

Figure 6.1. Profile of Essential Amino Acid Requirements. Protein quality is based on the amount of EAAs per gram of protein and how closely the profile of EAAs in the protein matches the profile of dietary requirements.

EAASE and the Dietary Guidelines

It is a fundamental premise of the EAASE program that the dietary guidelines are focused on minimal acceptable intake, and that the optimal amount and type of protein intake, as well as EAA intake, are not described by the RDAs or by the Dietary Guidelines for Americans. Throughout the rest of the book, I will share scientific findings and observations to convince you that "optimal EAA and protein nutrition" translates to a significantly higher intake of high quality protein and EAAs than the minimal standards recommended by the experts.

Essentials

- The Recommended Dietary Allowance (RDA) is defined to be the average daily nutrient intake level sufficient to meet the minimal nutrient requirement of nearly all healthy people.
- The protein RDA of 0.80 g protein intake/kg body weight/day (about 10% of caloric intake) is the minimum amount to maintain body nitrogen in healthy young adults.
- The DRIs recommend that up to 35% of energy intake be provided by protein.
- The average American consumes 1.2-1.5 g protein/kg body weight/day, which is about 20% of caloric intake. This is well within the range of protein intake recommended by the DRIs.
- There is an RDA for each individual EAA. Even as minimal values, the current EAA requirements are almost certainly too low for optimal nutrition. The optimal profile of EAAs in the diet will vary depending upon age, activity level and health conditions.
- Optimal protein nutrition demands greater intakes of protein and EAAs than the current RDAs.

Chapter 7. Dietary Protein

The RDA for protein corresponds to about 10 percent of daily caloric intake. As such, you might consider the protein content as a minor component of the diet. This perspective would be wrong. In fact, protein should take center stage in most every person's diet. There is a particularly good argument for the centrality of protein in an athlete's diet, in terms of both muscle mass and strength. More generally, dietary protein has a central role in the nutritional arsenal against the chronic diseases and stress many of us deal with every day. Many of these beneficial effects are also related to the effect of dietary protein on muscle. The starting point of the EAASE program is a balanced diet that contains the optimal amount of protein, rather than the minimal amount of dietary protein. I will first describe some of the reasons that eating the optimal amount of dietary protein is important.

Dietary protein is the only major nutrient that you have to eat to survive. Alaskan natives thrive on a diet of entirely protein and fat, and individuals who have had their intestines surgically removed can live for years on intravenous nutrition comprised almost entirely of amino acids and glucose, with only a very small amount of fat to meet the requirement for one specific fatty acid. That being said, you don't need to eat much dietary protein to satisfy the official recommendations discussed in the previous chapter. If you are eating a normal American diet, you are consuming more than the RDA for protein. Further, even if you eat low quality proteins that contain only a small amount of EAAs, you are probably eating enough above the RDA for protein to satisfy the RDAs for the EAAs as well. However, it is important to realize that the RDAs for protein and EAAs are the *minimal* amounts needed to avoid nutritional deficiencies. You can appreciate the minimal nature of the RDA for protein if you consider recommendations for protein in the context of the RDAs for all the major nutrients (i.e., carbohydrate, fat and protein). This approach makes sense, since the food we eat provides a mixture of these macronutrients (unless you are following an extreme type of diet). If you add up the caloric value of the sum total of the RDAs for dietary protein, carbohydrates and fat, it is less than half of the total amount of calories you need to eat each day to maintain energy balance (**Figure 7.1**).

94

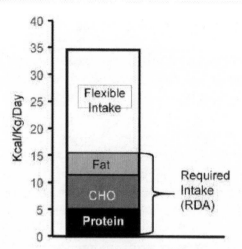

Figure 7.1. Required and flexible macronutrient intake. The RDAs for protein carbohydrate (CHO) and fat add up to about half of the calories we eat every day. The difference between the total amounts of calories you eat in a day as compared to the amount of calories you consume to meet the RDAs for the major nutrients can be considered as the flexible component of your diet. The flexible component of your diet consists of at least half of the calories you need to consume in the day. A significant part of your flexible daily caloric intake should be composed of protein foods. This point can be better appreciated if you consider the minimal vs optimal amount of daily consumption of protein.

Beneficial Effects of Dietary Proteins

Muscle Protein Turnover

When I was training for a competitive marathon, I could feel my muscles getting stronger as I ramped up my training. This was reflected in progressively faster times in interval training, such as running a hill multiple times in a workout, as well as continuous runs. However, I wasn't putting on muscle mass. I didn't want extra muscle, as the weight of more muscle would have required more work to sustain a fast running pace for two hours or more. The reason my muscles were getting stronger is that the "turnover" of muscle protein was increased by training. Muscle protein turnover refers to the breakdown of older proteins and synthesis of new proteins to replace the ones that were broken down. Increased muscle protein turnover improves muscle function because older, less efficient muscle fibers are replaced by better functioning newer fibers. Increased muscle protein turnover enables individual fibers to contract more efficiently and generate more force when they contract.

With endurance training, such as running or swimming, improvements in muscle function result not only from increased turnover of muscle fiber proteins, but also because of a greater ability to produce energy in the muscle. Training causes an increased number and capacity of the mitochondria in muscle. Mitochondria are the organelles in the cell that produce the energy that the muscle needs to contract during exercise. The reactions in the mitochondria that produce energy are made possible by a variety of proteins called *enzymes*. Increased turnover of mitochondrial proteins (i.e., the enzymes) is central to increases in the number and function of the mitochondria.

Dietary Protein and Muscle Protein Turnover

In outer space, the lack of gravity greatly reduces the difficulty of movement, and this reduces the demands on muscle.

Muscle thrives when forced to exercise, and doesn't do well when the physical demands are minimal. Since space flight reduces the demands on muscle, the loss of muscle mass and strength can be severe. One of the biggest concerns about flying to Mars is that the muscle loss would be so great that the crew could not continue to operate the space craft. The loss of muscle mass and particularly strength that occurs in space flight is due to a reduced rate of muscle protein turnover.

Dietary protein amplifies muscle protein turnover. This is true even at rest. We showed this in a series of studies we performed for NASA aimed at reducing the loss of muscle mass and function that occurs with space flight. To simulate the functional inactivity in space, we confined normal volunteers to strict bed rest for 28 days. During this time, the subjects could never leave the bed. Bed rest causes a loss of muscle mass and function similar to what occurs in space. When the level of protein consumption was increased 50% above the RDA for protein, the amount of muscle mass loss was significantly reduced because the normal reduction in protein turnover caused by bed rest was prevented by the increased protein intake.

Increased dietary protein also increases muscle protein turnover, and consequently both muscle mass and function, in free-living individuals. This effect is most evident in older individuals who may be eating an inadequate amount of protein. The effect of dietary protein on protein turnover is amplified by exercise. The stimulation of muscle protein turnover by exercise, per se, can only increase muscle protein turnover to a limited extent because of a shortage of the amino acid building blocks of protein. However, exercise "primes" the muscle to be more responsive to amino acids when they become available from the digestion of dietary protein. When resistance exercise and protein intake are combined, the increase in protein turnover not only improves muscle function as described above, but the rate of muscle protein synthesis may exceed the rate of breakdown, resulting in an increase in muscle mass. This is referred to as an *anabolic* response.

What Type of Protein Should We Eat?

Protein Quality

Eating an optimal amount of high quality protein is a cornerstone of the EAASE program. A high quality protein contains a high proportion of EAAs relative to the NEAAs. In addition, the profile of the EAAs, which is the amount of each EAA in relation to the others, is favorable in a high quality protein. The optimal profile is defined by the experts as closely paralleling the requirements for the individual EAAs. Also, the EAA in the dietary protein must be digested and absorbed into the body, and a high-quality protein is highly digestible. The Food and Agriculture Organization of The World Health Organization (FAO/WHO) is the official body that is responsible for coming up with a scoring system to rank the quality of dietary proteins. Some representative values are shown in **Figure 7.2**. The higher the quality of the protein, the higher the value.

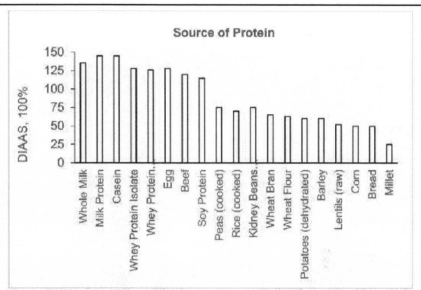

Figure 7.2. Ranking of the quality of some common foods. The quality of the protein calculated from the relation of the profile of each EAA relative to the profile of the corresponding EAA, the amount of EAAs per g of protein, and the digestibility of the protein. The score is called the Digestible Indispensable Amino Acid Score (DIAAS). A protein with a DIAAS of 100 or more is considered to be a high-quality protein.

The highest quality proteins are "animal" based or derived from animals; these include meat, dairy, fish, poultry and eggs. Lower quality proteins include many of the plant-based proteins like those in wheat, beans, and rice. They are lower quality because they do not provide adequate amounts of all the EAAs and because of poorer digestibility and absorption.

Protein Food Sources

When thinking about the values shown in Figure 7.2, it probably occurs to you that, except in the case of protein supplements, we don't eat purified proteins. Rather, we eat them in food sources. There are a number of things to consider when evaluating a protein food source. In addition to the protein quality, we should think about the non-protein components of the protein food source. For example, when you eat a steak you are consuming a lot of high quality protein, but you are also eating some saturated fat. When you eat kidney beans as a protein food source, you are also eating carbohydrate and fiber. These factors should be taken into account in dietary planning.

The *protein density* is high in a high quality protein food source. Protein density refers to the amount of protein per total grams of food source. The significance of protein density can be appreciated by looking at the number of calories that must be consumed from a protein food source to meet all daily EAA requirements. **Figure 7.3** presents some representative values.

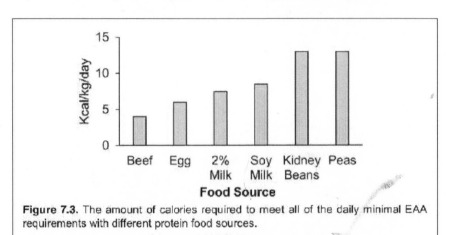

Figure 7.3. The amount of calories required to meet all of the daily minimal EAA requirements with different protein food sources.

You may find some values surprising. For example, the hamburger is the poster-child for why Americans are fat, yet the number of calories you consume in the form of a beef patty to obtain all of your EAA requirements for the day is less than one-third the amount of calories you need if you look to plant-based proteins to meet your EAA requirements. Further, the fiber in plant-based food sources, while providing some health benefits, at the same time further impedes the digestion of the EAAs in the protein component of the food.

Whether you look at protein quality scores, or the protein density of protein food sources it is evident why consumption of a variety of animal-based proteins simplifies the task of satisfying EAA requirements. It is possible to achieve adequate protein/EAA nutrition on a vegetarian or even a vegan diet, but much more careful planning of your dietary pattern is necessary. This planning is important because you will consume a much higher proportion of your caloric allotment for the day in conjunction with your protein food source, and this leaves less flexibility for the remainder of your diet. EAA supplements play a crucial role in enabling you to achieve optimal EAA nutrition in all circumstances, but this is particularly true if you rely on plant-based protein food sources.

Complementary Dietary Proteins

Figure 7.3 shows how many calories will be consumed in order to meet all of the EAA requirements if that is the only food source you eat. However, we eat a variety of protein food sources every day, and there is potential for complementary proteins to provide a complete profile of EAAs even if each one is deficient on its own. This matching is of real importance in a vegetarian diet. It is theoretically possible to make up for the poor quality of plant-based protein food sources by eating complementary proteins. The idea is to match protein food sources that are deficient in different amino acids and the combination of the two or more will meet all EAA requirements. In the southern part of the United States, the combination of red beans and rice is popular and is often cited as a good example of complementary proteins. The idea is that while neither is a high quality protein food source, together they provide a more balanced mixture of EAAs.

There are many examples of complementary proteins working synergistically in a diet to provide a good balance of EAAs. However, there are a few things about complementary proteins that you should keep in mind. First, they have to be eaten at the same time. All the EAAs must be increased at the same time and in the appropriate profile to fully stimulate protein synthesis. Second, and most importantly, they must have truly complementary profiles of EAAs. The quality of most plant-based proteins is limited by the availability of lysine. Therefore, it is unlikely that two plant-based proteins will be truly complementary. This is in fact the case with red beans and rice, for example. The combination of red beans and rice go together nicely in a meal, but the concept that they are complementary proteins is more legend than fact. Also, if the two food sources are both low quality proteins, the total amount of calories that will be consumed to meet EAA requirements with those food sources will be quite significant.

In contrast to the difficulty of finding complementary plant-based proteins, a typical omnivore diet, combining animal protein and plant-based protein foods is quite effective. Matching proteins that have different limiting EAAs is much easier. It is also very effective to use nutrient supplementation with EAAs in combination with low quality plant-based protein food sources to improve the overall diet quality. This approach will be discussed when I give the details of the EAASE program.

Fast vs Slow Proteins

Proteins must be digested to their component amino acids before the amino acids can be absorbed into the body. This process is surprisingly variable in its efficiency, and the quality of the protein is impacted by the efficiency of the digestive process. In addition, the digestion time varies considerably between proteins. For example, whey protein and casein are the primary proteins in milk. The whey protein component is digested very rapidly while the casein is digested very slowly. This combination makes milk protein an effective source of protein. Not only is the amount and profile of EAAs favorable, but the digestion of the protein starts fast (whey) and lasts over an extended period of time (casein).

The importance of the speed of digestion in terms of the stimulation of muscle protein synthesis was recently demonstrated by an experiment done by a group of investigators in Canada. They gave a dose of whey protein as a single shot or divided the same amount of whey protein into 5 portions consumed over 4 hours. The single dose elicited a greater response of muscle protein synthesis even though the same exact amount of whey protein was given in the two different patterns. This study showed the importance of the rapid absorption of the amino acids resulting from the digestion of the protein. The key seemed to be that the peak concentrations of EAAs reached with the entire dose consumed in one shot was much higher than when presented in a way to mimic a "slow" protein digestion (like casein).

The rapid absorption of the amino acids in dietary proteins is important because the EAAs reach peak concentrations that are higher than is the case with a slow protein. In addition, if the protein supplement is consumed between meals, a slow protein may still be in the process of being digested when the next meal is eaten. The active digestion of a protein coinciding with consumption of the next meal is likely to diminish the normal anabolic effect of the meal, as well as blunt the appetite. The latter response can be used to your advantage during caloric restriction weight loss, but is not a desirable response in most circumstances.

Bioavailability of Nutrients

Complete protein food sources provide not only macronutrients, they also contain many vitamins, minerals and other nutrients (*micronutrients*). To understand how much of a given micronutrient from food actually enters the body, we need to think about *bioavailability*. Bioavailability refers to the proportion of a substance that enters the circulation after it is consumed. Bioavailability of iron is a good example familiar to many people. Red meat is a good source of iron and spinach is also promoted as a good source of iron (just think of Popeye the Sailor). When compared with red meat, spinach contains almost the same amount: 100 g of spinach contains 2.7 mg of iron versus 2.6 mg found in 100 g of meat. But the difference is that iron from animal foods has a higher absorption in the body than the iron from plant/vegetable sources. To obtain the same amount of iron found in a three-ounce serving of beef, you'd have to eat at least three cups of raw spinach. Dietary recommendations in the EAASE program have taken account of bioavailability in the recommendations of protein food sources.

Sustainability of the Environment and Protein Food Sources

It is clear from a factual basis that animal-based protein food sources provide higher quality proteins in a nutrient-dense package relative to plant-based proteins. However, there is a movement to decrease the consumption of animal-based protein because animals contribute to the carbon production that is purportedly causing global warming. It is not a lunatic fringe that promotes eliminating animal-based protein from the diet on the basis of saving the world. The 2015 scientific report of the Dietary Guidelines for Americans articulated this position. Since eating high quality animal protein is part of the EAASE program, it is reasonable to address this legitimate concern.

The environmental issues raised against animal protein food sources are based on carbon production, in the form of CO_2 and methane (primarily from cows). Before making an informed decision on eliminating animal protein from our diet, other factors should also be considered. First, animals such as cattle and sheep are remarkably efficient- they consume grass, which has no nutritional value to humans, and convert it into the highest quality protein. Second, most pasture land throughout the world cannot be used to grow crops. Third, the requirements to produce sufficient plant-based proteins to adequately substitute for the elimination of animal protein from our diet must be considered. These requirements include not only the space, but water availability, fertilizer and a very large amount of equipment that must be produced and operated to farm vast numbers of crops. Until these factors are adequately addressed, it is premature to advocate eliminating animal proteins from our diet on the basis of environmental considerations.

While the above arguments should console those of you who feel guilty about eating a good steak, I fully recognize that many people opt to not eat animal protein, either because of the environmental issues or other concerns. For those of you who have chosen this path, it is important to understand the concepts discussed in this chapter regarding protein quality. It is possible to achieve optimal EAA nutrition with a vegan diet, but doing so will almost certainly require including an EAA supplement in your normal daily diet.

- Calories provided by foods to meet the RDAs for protein, carbohydrate and fat totals less than half of the average person's total caloric requirement. The remainder of caloric intake to meet energy needs can be considered flexible.
- Dietary protein should comprise a significant portion of the flexible caloric intake.
- Protein quality is determined by the amount and profile of EAAs, as well as digestibility of the protein.
- Protein food sources contain not only the protein, but non-protein calories as well. The total calories that will be consumed to meet EAA requirements are higher with food sources containing low quality (as opposed to high quality) dietary proteins.
- Eating complementary proteins can compensate for deficiencies of low quality proteins. The combination of an animal protein and plant-based food source can be effective, but plant-based proteins that are limited by the same amino acid do not form a complementary pair.
- Bioavailability refers to the extent to which the nutrient in a food source enters the blood.
- Issues of sustainability of the environment or concern for animal welfare may prompt some to eliminate animal-based protein from the diet. There are many practical issues to consider regarding the feasibility of producing enough plant protein foods to replace the unique characteristics and quality of animal-based proteins.
- A diet relying on plant-based protein requires careful planning to account for the relatively low content of EAAs in the dietary protein. The use of EAA supplements can compensate for the low EAA content of the regular diet, thereby achieving optimal EAA nutrition.

Chapter 8. Protein and Amino Acid Supplements

Supplements vs Whole Foods

A number of years ago, I was part of an advisory group to the International Olympic Committee charged with making dietary guidelines for Olympic athletes in different sports. There was an interesting discussion at the outset of the deliberations when one of the members of the committee made the proposal that the overriding dietary recommendation would be that nutrients should be obtained from eating whole foods rather than dietary supplements. The discussion that followed focused on practical issues, such as the fact that many athletes lived in group housing or other circumstances in which they had little control over the meals they were served, and that long training hours often caused athletes to miss serving hours. In those days, Olympic athletes were true amateurs, and cost and preparation time was often a factor limiting food choices. There was little consideration of the possibility that dietary supplements could provide specific nutrients more effectively than any natural food.

The problems faced by elite athletes in obtaining quality, healthy diets became abundantly clear to me when I lived in Santa Barbara in the early1970's. Santa Barbara had become a center for track and field athletes training for international competition because of the perfect year-round weather, and the excellent training facilities. However, there was no "training table" available to these athletes. Instead, many of the athletes figured out the schedule of which nights the local bars served free hors d'oeuvres during happy hour. While chips and dip and chicken wings might be tasty treats, they would hardly constitute a great diet for athletes training for the Olympics. It was obvious that dietary supplements had to be a central part of their nutrient intake, and to recommend a diet of only whole foods missed the reality of how athletes lived at that time.

A lot has changed since the 1970's with regard to our diets. There has been a vast amount of research into what a healthy diet looks like, and there has been a concerted effort to pass this information along to the general public. On the other hand, the abundance of cheap and quick food choices is, in many cases, at odds with "healthy" diets. Further, that which we are told is a "healthy" diet by the experts is more and more influenced by political issues rather than the results of solid scientific studies. As a result, the incidence of nutrition-related health issues has escalated drastically since the 1970's, most prominently obesity and diabetes. The older population in particular is vulnerable to problems related to nutrition. Obesity is a common problem in older individuals, which limits mobility and adversely impacts quality of life. At the same time, undernutrition occurs in as much as 30% of the population of individuals over the age of 65 years. Undernutrition contributes to the loss of muscle mass and strength that occurs with aging, and this can progress to the point where the ability to perform activities of daily living is limited. This problem has become so pervasive in the elderly that is has been given its own name-*sarcopenia*. In alarming numbers, the occurrence of sarcopenia and obesity are occurring simultaneously, creating what is termed *sarcopenic obesity*. Individuals with sarcopenic obesity must move a large and heavy mass of fat with a depleted muscle mass.

All of the nutritional challenges facing us today have made the problems of the athletes of the 1970's getting proper nutrition seem trivial. While consumption of healthy whole foods will always be a central part of any reasonable nutrition plan, the role of nutritional supplements in balancing the nutritional needs of the entire population has never been greater. With particular relevance to the EAASE program, dietary supplements of EAAs have a clear place in enabling better amino acid and protein nutrition than possible with natural food alone.

Challenges of Nutritional Supplements

The enormous growth in the field of nutritional supplements reflects the overwhelming desire of people to consume important nutrients that they might be missing in their diet. Unfortunately, the consumer is bombarded with information that can be difficult to sort out. Most often, claims are unsupported by scientific studies, and may be at odds with basic physiology. This has led to a general disdain of nutritional supplements by the traditional medical community. This is why the EAASE program is based entirely on studies published in highly-reviewed scientific journals. The most relevant of these studies are listed in the Bibliography. My goal is to deliver a program in the context of the physiology of the body. If you understand the very basic concepts presented, you can appreciate the validity and importance of each specific component of the EAASE Program.

Protein Supplements

Dietary supplements containing protein have become ubiquitous. They come in all shapes and formats - powders, bars, beverages, etc. These supplements can provide a good boost to your daily protein intake, but there are a few things that can limit the value of protein supplements. In the previous chapter, I discussed protein quality being determined by the amount and profile of the EAAs. Unfortunately, the highest quality proteins are usually the most expensive, and may have taste and food-science issues such as solubility and texture that make the production of a flavorful and inexpensive supplement difficult. Lower quality proteins may be used to get around some of the issues raised by using high-quality proteins. Collagen is a very popular component of protein supplements because it is cheap, soluble, and does not have an unpleasant taste. Unfortunately, collagen is a very low quality protein that has a low and unbalanced proportion of EAAs. Soy protein is also commonly used in supplements, and it has the highest content of EAAs of the vegetable proteins (but less than animal proteins). However, some soy formulations also contain a substance called genistein that has widespread effects in the body, including binding to the estrogen receptors and exerting estrogen-like effects. Estrogen is identified as a feminizing hormone, not typically the effect people are seeking with a protein supplement.

Recently, other vegetable proteins have become popular components of protein-enriched products. For example, pea protein is being used more commonly in supplements. Although peas are a poor source of protein because of the small amount of protein per pea, if the protein is isolated in pure form, it is not a bad source of EAAs and it is cheap.

Whey protein is the most popular protein supplement. Whey protein is a milk protein that is a by-product of the production of cheese. It is a high quality protein with an excellent content and profile of EAAs. Whey protein is not a single protein, but is composed of a variety of proteins and peptides (short chains of amino acids). In the form in which whey is separated during cheese production, whey contains more carbohydrate than protein. The carbohydrates are partly lactose which induces an adverse response in individuals who are lactose intolerant. Whey protein isolate is produced by further processing of natural whey protein, and results in a product that has as much as 90% protein, with the rest mainly composed of carbohydrates. The addition of flavoring to whey protein isolate may add up to 30% additional carbohydrates. The important point is that whey protein, similar to all other protein supplements and protein food sources is not pure protein.

Labeling of Protein Supplement Products

The discerning customer knows what he or she wants. The information provided about a product is often limited to the label on the package and, unfortunately, the labels can range from uninformative to downright deceptive. For example, it is not unusual for "pure whey protein" to contain as little as 60% of calories as whey protein, with the balance of calories being comprised of carbohydrate and fat. The lesson is: buyer beware-don't just buy on the basis of the name of a product, but dig into what the product actually provides.

Another labeling issue that is of considerable concern is trying to figure out the relative proportions of different proteins in a mixture of proteins. Most supplements include some whey protein, as it is widely accepted as one of the highest quality proteins. However, because of cost, and certain characteristics, other proteins are often included in a mixture with whey protein. Soy and collagen are the most commonly included proteins in a mixture. Labeling rarely includes the proportion of each protein. Consequently, the true protein quality of the protein contained in some supplements is uncertain. Ingredients are listed in order of descending quantity so the first ingredient listed is ideally a high quality protein.

Finally, it is the right of consumers to expect that what they are consuming is what they believe it to be. Spot-checking of nutritional supplements has often revealed that the actual contents do not match the labelling. Interestingly, it can happen that something not mentioned on the label is actually included. For this reason, it is advisable to only buy supplements whose contents have been certified by an independent source such as US Pharmacopeia, or to at least check the web page of the producer to determine if they have the appropriate certifications. This issue is of particular concern for athletes who could be unwittingly consuming banned substances. Numerous cases of positive tests for banned substances have occurred as a consequence of the inclusion of something in a supplement that was not mentioned in the packaging. Although it may seem unfair, this is not an excuse for a positive test. Although the industry has been making progress in cleaning up this problem, it still persists. Protein supplements are not regulated by the Food and Drug Administration, so the responsibility falls on the consumer to deal only with reputable suppliers.

Amino Acids as Supplements

Free amino acid supplements offer potential advantages as compared with protein supplements in several respects. Most importantly, amino acid mixtures can be formulated exactly as desired. Precise mixtures of amino acids can thus be produced that target specific metabolic issues. In addition, free amino acids can be completely absorbed more rapidly than any intact protein. After ingestion of a mixture of free EAAs, the corresponding peak concentrations are higher and are achieved more rapidly than even the response to whey protein. Whey protein is a "fast" protein, meaning that it is digested and absorbed very rapidly as compared to other dietary proteins. In the previous chapter, I discussed the benefit of a "fast" vs "slow" protein in terms of the stimulation of protein synthesis, and free amino acids surpass the absorption characteristics of even the "fastest" protein. The result is that the metabolic response to free EAAs often surpasses the maximal effect that can be achieved with intact protein, and often with a smaller dose.

The advantages of free EAA mixtures can be seen in the comparison of the response of muscle protein synthesis to different doses of a balanced mixture of all the free EAAs as compared to whey protein and to a partial mixture of only BCAAs. The extent of stimulation of muscle protein synthesis by different doses of EAAs as compared to BCAAs and whey protein is shown in **Figure 8.1**.

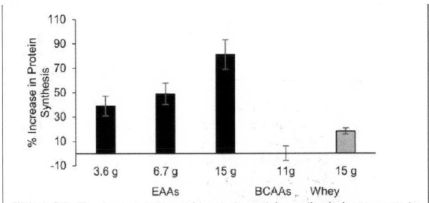

Figure 8.1. The percent increase in muscle protein synthesis in response to different doses of EAAs, BCAAs, or whey protein. Whey protein is the most effective intact protein.

Dietary proteins are made up of a range of amino acids including both EAAs and NEAAs. Consequently, intact protein supplements cannot target a specific amino-acid related metabolic response. In contrast, the use of single free amino acid supplements is a simple solution to target the intake of a specific amino acid for a desired outcome. A single amino acid supplement will increase the blood concentration of that particular amino acid but the magnitude and duration of the increase will vary depending upon the starting concentration of the amino acid. For example, the amount of tyrosine circulating in the blood is quite small, so ingestion of a small amount of tyrosine may increase the plasma concentration significantly, while consumption of the same amount of alanine, which is normally abundant in plasma, will have minimal effect on the plasma concentration.

In theory, the use of a single amino acid supplement may elicit a desired response, but oftentimes, this is not the case. Also, while the targeted response may be positively affected, other responses may not be desirable. If you think about the human body at work, all day and night and every day and night, there are a multitude of physiological events taking place at the same time. While the stomach is digesting food and the intestines are absorbing nutrients, the liver is at work processing carbohydrates, fats and amino acids. The muscles are moving, the heart is pumping blood, the lungs are breathing, and the brain is sending signals to control everything. Underlying these major functions are countless chemical reactions and continuous breakdown and synthesis of compounds, all needed to sustain these vital organs and to sustain life. All of these functions require a balanced supply of amino acids, which is disrupted by the excess consumption of a single, or limited mixture, of amino acids. A balanced mixture of EAAs will provide the least disruption of the overall balance of the plasma amino acids while targeting specific metabolic reactions.

The Importance of Having All of the EAAs

Amino acids play a role, either directly or indirectly, in nearly every physiological function. Each amino acid serves multiple purposes and often works in concert with other amino acids. The simultaneous action of amino acids in a wide variety of reactions and functions helps to explain the nutritional value of a balanced mixture of all the EAAs. A major advantage of mixtures of EAAs is that many metabolic circumstances dictate an optimal profile of dietary amino acids that cannot be met by naturally occurring proteins. The utilization and functioning of individual amino acids is dependent upon many other conditions beyond simple supply and demand. The most important thing to remember is that although you may be taking an amino acid supplement for a specific purpose, all the other functions of amino acids continue. I will discuss some specific examples using claims made for various amino acid supplements to illustrate the interaction of EAAs, and how any nutritional supplementation that disrupts the overall balance of EAAs in an unanticipated way may have adverse effects.

Methionine and Cysteine Supplementation

The sulfur-containing amino acids methionine and cysteine are an example of how the action of one amino acid is affected by the other. Early findings on the effect of sulfur-containing amino acids on liver fat were confusing. In general, methionine was found to lower liver fat while cysteine seemed to promote fatty liver. In 1944, an investigator found that methionine supplementation could result in fatty liver when low protein diets were fed to the animals. Eventually, it was understood that a proper balance in the ratio of methionine to cysteine was necessary to maintain liver health and function.

Amino Acids and Brain Neurotransmitters

Another example of the importance of a balance in EAA concentrations involves the role of certain amino acids as brain neurotransmitters. The particular balance of amino acids that serve as precursors of neurotransmitters will influence brain-related functions since there is a competitive transport system for amino acids to get into the brain thus favoring amino acids present in the highest concentrations.

Leucine Supplementation and Muscle Protein Synthesis

A dietary supplement of leucine alone will increase the intracellular concentration in muscle effectively and may have the intended effect of activating the intracellular signaling involved in the initiation of muscle protein synthesis. At the same time, increasing leucine concentration intracellularly will activate the enzyme that degrades leucine as well as valine and isoleucine. The result is that leucine increases less than you might expect from the amount given, and the intracellular concentrations of valine and isoleucine will fall. The imbalance in all the EAAs resulting from the consumption of leucine alone will offset any beneficial effects of leucine on activating the initiation of protein synthesis.

Taken together, these examples are meant to highlight the fact that the optimal amino acid supplement must not only target a specific intended metabolic response, but also account for all other aspects of the physiological state and metabolic reactions related to the supplement.

BCAAs (leucine, isoleucine and valine) constitute about 35% of the EAAs in muscle protein. Furthermore, leucine seems to play a unique role as a regulator of muscle protein synthesis by activating molecular factors involved in the initiation of protein synthesis. For those reasons, BCAA supplements are currently quite popular. However, as discussed above, BCAAs alone do not stimulate muscle protein synthesis, and in fact the few studies measuring the response to BCAAs have shown a decreased rate of muscle protein synthesis. The response to BCAA ingestion, and in particular leucine, provides a good example of the circumstance in which an "activating" amino acid needs other amino acids present. There is no doubt from molecular studies that leucine can "turn on" the muscle protein synthetic machinery by activating factors in the initiation phase of this process. However, the activation of these initiation factors does not always result in the making of muscle protein because all of the amino acids are required to actually synthesize muscle in living beings. Leucine can be thought of as "the key to the car" which can start it up but fuel is still required in the tank to proceed further.

EAA Supplements

The preceding information makes a good argument for the benefit of creating effective free amino acid supplements using balanced amino acid mixtures that take account not only of the individual roles of specific amino acids but also the overall physiological response. After a month of fasting, plasma EAA levels are still maintained at the same level as an overnight fast. This observation indicates that keeping a balanced profile of amino acids in the blood is a high metabolic priority. Conceptually, this suggests that dietary supplements that disrupt the normal profile of all EAAs work against the natural regulation of amino acid metabolism. Following this logic, consumption of a single amino acid supplement or supplements containing a few EAAs would be undesirable except in condition-specific cases of an isolated deficiency. A more balanced approach to amino acid supplementation will enable the benefits of particular amino acids to be achieved in the context of more desirable physiological circumstances.

Balanced amino acid mixtures are available as supplements, most commonly sold as capsules, typically containing 500 mg of amino acids per capsule. Powdered flavored beverage mixtures offer the advantage of delivering the effective dose (minimum dose for affecting muscle metabolism is 3.0 g) in one serving rather than multiple capsules (typically 6 or more). Consuming amino acids in the free form provides the advantage of rapid absorption and complete bioavailability. Since only EAAs are needed for protein synthesis, EAA supplements provide an extra benefit since they promote recycling of the circulating non-essential amino acids back into protein. The advantage of leaving NEAAs out of a supplement to stimulate muscle protein synthesis is that the circulating NEAAs will be used more efficiently, rather than being metabolized to urea and ammonia. Leucine concentration can be boosted in these mixtures in order to maximize molecular signaling which may help overcome situations of anabolic resistance. Simultaneously, providing sufficient amounts of the other EAAs will allow the activation of synthesis to be reflected in increased muscle building.

It is important to recognize that not all EAA supplements are the same. The amino acids may be derived either from vegan or non-vegan sources. Amino acids from either source are equally effective physiologically, but the source may be a consideration if you are following a specific diet. More importantly, the profile of EAA formulations may differ. The effectiveness of any particular formulation of EAAs can only be known from research performed using the defined formulation in the specific physiological circumstance intended for use.

- Contemporary nutrition-related concerns include obesity and diabetes. The role of nutrition in athletic competition is also becoming more widely recognized.
- The elderly suffer from undernutrition, sarcopenia (loss of muscle), and sarcopenic obesity (loss of muscle occurring in an obese individual).
- Protein supplements are very popular and many products utilizing a wide variety of proteins are available.
- Whey is a milk protein composed of a variety of proteins and peptides. The amount of whey protein in a supplement varies widely with different processing methods.
- Supplement consumers should read nutrition labels carefully and try to select supplements manufactured by certified companies.
- Amino acids in blood and tissues are normally maintained at tightly-regulated concentrations and their functions are dependent on the balance of amino acids available.
- Individual amino acid supplements will increase blood concentration of that particular amino acid, but the magnitude and duration of the increase will vary depending upon the concentration of the amino acid in the blood.
- Proper amino acid functioning in the body is dependent on the balance of amino acids. An excess or a deficit of one amino acid can influence the amount and/or activity of another amino acid.
- Free amino acid supplements may be beneficial in condition-specific circumstances, keeping in mind that interactions occur between amino acids, and that data supporting the value of single amino acid supplements is sparse.
- Formulations of a complete and balanced nature are more efficient since they can be formulated to target specific metabolic reactions in the context of an overall beneficial physiological effect.

Chapter 9. Exercise

Aerobic Exercise

Aerobic exercise generally refers to activities that can be sustained for a significant period of time, such as jogging, biking and swimming. The term *aerobic* implies that there is enough oxygen available at the tissue level to supply all that is needed to perform the exercise. If the intensity increases beyond your capacity to deliver enough oxygen to the muscle to fully meet demand, the exercise is termed *anaerobic*. You can't sustain anaerobic exercise for very long-it would usually be the finishing sprint of a race, or a supra-maximal effort like running a 100 meter dash. Aerobic exercise is often used interchangeably with endurance exercise, but technically they are not necessarily the same because endurance exercise may have a component that is not aerobic.

Substrate Metabolism during Aerobic Exercise

The focus of this book is amino acid and protein metabolism, but when talking about the physiological response to aerobic exercise, a brief background regarding what substrates the muscle uses for energy is directly relevant to amino acid and protein metabolism. Substrate refers to the fuel used by the body. The majority of energy for exercising muscle is derived from the metabolism of either carbohydrate or fat.

Carbohydrate in the body is either in the form of glucose circulating in the blood or glycogen stored in the muscle or liver. Glycogen is the storage form of glucose. It consists of many glucose molecules hooked together. The glycogen stored in muscle can be directly used for energy, and muscle can also tap the glycogen in the liver by extracting glucose from the circulating blood. As the muscle extracts glucose from the blood, glycogen is converted back to glucose in the liver. This glucose is then released into the blood to maintain the plasma glucose level constant. Insulin is a hormone that aids in the uptake of glucose by muscle.

Fat is stored in the body as triglycerides. Triglycerides consist of three fatty acids linked together. Triglycerides in fat tissue can be broken down and the free fatty acids released into the blood, and the muscle can take up the circulating free fatty acids to use for the production of energy to fuel exercise. In addition, triglyceride is stored in muscle, and that source of potential energy can be used by exercising muscle as well.

The balance between the uses of these different potential sources of energy for exercising muscle depends on the intensity of the exercise and the level of training. Low intensity exercise, like jogging or easy cycling, relies mainly on circulating fatty acids for energy. This is why low intensity exercise is referred to as the "fat burning" zone, and why low-intensity exercise is advocated if you are trying to lose fat. Carbohydrate usage in the form of muscle glycogen becomes more prominent as the exercise intensity increases. Once muscle glycogen is depleted, the muscle must rely almost entirely on fatty acids for energy. Only highly trained individuals have adapted the pathways of fatty acid metabolism sufficiently to maintain a high level of performance once muscle glycogen is depleted. The point at which muscle glycogen is depleted is often described as "hitting the wall".

Training has a significant impact on the nature of substrate metabolism during exercise. Training increases the ability to use fat as an energy source. Increased reliance on fatty acids delays the depletion of muscle glycogen and "hitting the wall".

125

Since the depletion of muscle glycogen impairs performance in all but highly trained endurance athletes, carbohydrate-based energy supplements have gained enormous popularity. The theory is that, when consumed during exercise, energy supplements (usually in the form of beverages) can provide a significant source of energy for muscle, and thereby spare the muscle glycogen and prolong the time until the muscle glycogen is depleted. Carbohydrate-based energy supplements are advocated after exercise to replete the muscle glycogen used during exercise.

Despite the enormous popularity of carbohydrate-based energy beverages, the benefits of these products are quite limited in most circumstances. If you are exercising at a high enough intensity to rely on stored glycogen in muscle, you are using fuel at such a fast rate that the amount you can ingest while exercising is only a small fraction of what you need. Furthermore, if you drink glucose while exercising, it will inhibit the rate of fatty acid oxidation. One of the primary goals of training, whether for the Olympic marathon or just to try to gain a little fitness, is to amplify the ability to oxidize fatty acids, so you are countering this adaptive response by drinking a carbohydrate-based beverage. This explains why for many, it is best to be in a post-absorptive state when you do your training, since this will maximize reliance on fatty acids as sources of energy.

Following exercise, it is important to restore your muscle glycogen. However, even though you may feel tired after a workout, you probably have not depleted your muscle glycogen. It takes between an hour and one and a half hours to deplete your muscle glycogen when continuously exercising at 70% of your maximal capacity. While an athlete may do this routinely, recreational athletes are rarely capable of doing this kind of training on a regular basis. For most, post-exercise sports beverage consumption does not have to target repletion of muscle glycogen as a priority.

While the majority of energy for exercise comes from carbohydrates and fats, the oxidation of leucine also increases during exercise. This is a selective response, as the oxidation of other EAAs is not increased (**Figure 9.1**).

(margin handwriting: INCREASES BY 250%. TRIPLINK FROM BASAL RATE)

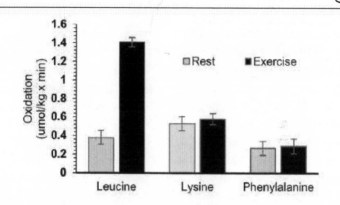

Figure 9.1. Leucine, lysine and phenylalanine oxidation during aerobic exercise. Leucine oxidation increased 3-fold above the basal rate during exercise at 60% of maximal capacity, while other EAAs, represented by lysine and phenylalanine in the figure, did not change significantly.

(margin handwriting: LEUCINE IS ONLY 1%.)

Even with a threefold increase in leucine oxidation during exercise, it is not a significant contributor to total energy production. The oxidation of leucine contributed a total of 8 μmole CO_2/kg/min to the total rate of CO_2 production while fatty acid oxidation contributed 828 μmole/kg/min. Although not quantitatively important in terms of total energy production, the metabolism of the EAAs during exercise is important in two respects.

First, the selective metabolism of leucine during exercise reduces its concentration in blood. An imbalance in the EAA concentrations in blood is always a problem in terms of the synthesis of new proteins. Also, there is a theory that leucine depletion can induce fatigue. The theory is called the "central fatigue hypothesis". If you recall from the discussion of neurotransmitters in the overview of the brain, amino acids serve as the building blocks for certain neurotransmitters. Tryptophan is an EAA that is converted into serotonin in the brain. Tryptophan and leucine are structurally similar and therefore, compete for the same transporter to get into the brain. When the blood concentration of leucine falls during prolonged aerobic exercise, more tryptophan enters the brain and the amount of serotonin is increased. Serotonin is an inhibitory neurotransmitter, which means that it suppresses nerve cell firing and amplifies the feeling of fatigue. Some people believe that "central fatigue" explains why we tire during endurance exercise even though a physiological steady state exists. Even in more moderate activities like golf, it is suggested that supplemental leucine or BCAAs can minimize serotonin activity and help in maintaining "mental focus" for the many hours of the golf round. It is hard to quantify "mental focus", so the central fatigue hypothesis has not been proven but remains intriguing.

The second important aspect of the accelerated oxidation of the leucine during exercise is that it impacts protein turnover, particularly in muscle. Both aerobic and resistance exercise accelerate muscle protein turnover meaning that both synthesis and breakdown are increased. The initial response to exercise is the breakdown of muscle which increases the availability of free EAAs. These EAAs, in turn, stimulate new muscle protein synthesis. The increased turnover of muscle protein results in newer, better-functioning proteins replacing the older muscle fibers that are not as efficient in generating force when they contract during exercise. However, if leucine is oxidized for energy during prolonged exercise, then it is no longer available to be reincorporated into muscle. If the body doesn't have all the building blocks necessary to make muscle, the beneficial effect of exercise on muscle will be limited.

EAA Supplements and Aerobic Exercise

Are there any benefits to consuming EAA or BCAA supplements before aerobic exercise? Since leucine (and probably isoleucine and valine, although that hasn't been measured) can be used for energy during endurance exercise, it may seem reasonable to supply extra leucine or BCAAs as a supplement to prevent the oxidation of BCAAs that come from muscle breakdown. Remember though, that when you give more leucine or BCAAs, a greater percentage is oxidized. The efficiency of the supplement is therefore considerably reduced when given before or during aerobic exercise when the metabolic pathways of BCAA oxidation are already revved up. Consequently, the supplemental leucine or BCAAs will not be available to promote muscle protein turnover.

In contrast to the circumstance before or during exercise, an EAA supplement (but not BCAA supplement) can provide great benefit if taken in the first hour after aerobic exercise. EAAs supply the precursors for protein synthesis to fuel an increase in protein turnover. An increase in muscle protein turnover is the metabolic basis for improved muscle fiber functioning. In addition, the EAAs will increase the production and functioning of the mitochondria, which is the site in the cell where energy is produced. These responses can only be achieved with a formulation containing all of the EAAs. While BCAAs alone are not effective, the optimal EAA formulation for post-exercise supplementation should have a higher proportion of BCAAs in the total mixture than represented in the composition of muscle protein in order to restore what was metabolized during exercise.

Resistance Exercise

Muscle Strength vs Muscle Mass

Resistance training can take many forms, but you are probably most familiar with lifting weights or using machines in a gym. Increasing muscle strength is a primary goal of resistance exercise. <u>Muscle strength does not necessarily require an increase in muscle mass.</u> Also, increasing muscle mass may or may not be your goal. I can personally relate to the different goals you might have with weight training. When I was competing in basketball, I wanted to get stronger, and I also wanted to get bigger so I wouldn't be pushed around as easily. When I started training seriously for marathons, my goals with resistance exercise changed. Extra body weight is a liability to a distance runner- my weight when I was a serious distance runner was 20 lbs lighter than when I played basketball. Nonetheless, during long runs my arms and shoulders would get fatigued and tighten up, so I wanted to increase my arm strength without increasing my weight. Even if your goal is to get bigger, there are different perspectives. If you are a lineman for a football team or participating in a power sport such as shot putting, you want increased strength and mass, and particularly function. If you are body-building, you want to increase muscle protein mass, but also minimize body fat and muscle glycogen in order to get the "ripped" look. Just as your training will differ, depending on the desired result, so too will the optimal nutrition, including EAA supplements.

Resistance Exercise and Protein Turnover

Increasing muscle strength and mass requires a close interaction between the exercise, regular diet, and EAA supplementation. Resistance exercise stimulates muscle protein turnover. This is how muscle fiber function improves. Newer, better functioning fibers are synthesized to replace older ones that are not functioning as well. Both muscle protein breakdown and protein synthesis are stimulated. Resistance exercise increases the efficiency of protein synthesis, so the increase in synthesis will be slightly greater than the increase in breakdown. The stimulation of protein synthesis is limited, however, because some of the EAAs released by protein breakdown are oxidized and not available for synthesis. Thus, even though the muscle is able to produce new protein more efficiently, the balance between muscle protein synthesis and breakdown remains negative (i.e., net loss of muscle protein) in the absence of nutrient intake. Resistance exercise does not result in a positive muscle protein balance if you are a power lifter and perform only two or three lifts of maximal exertion in a workout, or if you are a distance runner and doing 30 repetitions of a lift to tone and strengthen muscle. You must consume EAAs to at least balance those oxidized during the exercise to result in a net increase in muscle mass.

Protein Turnover and EAAs

The persistence of the net breakdown of muscle protein during and after resistance exercise can only be reversed by ingestion of nutrients, specifically EAAs. If an EAA supplement is ingested 30 minutes before resistance exercise, the muscle is put into a very anabolic state. If the EAAs are consumed immediately after the exercise there is also a stimulation of net muscle protein synthesis, but less than if given before the workout (**Figure 9.2**). The importance of taking the EAAs before the workout is that the net breakdown of muscle protein during the workout will be prevented. In part this is because the increase in blood flow to the muscle during the exercise will deliver the ingested amino acids to the muscle. By increasing the blood concentrations of EAAs, the concentration gradients will force EAAs into the muscle cells instead of out, which is the case without EAA supplementation. Consuming EAAs after the workout will further stimulate protein synthesis and prolong the anabolic response. The optimal approach is to take EAAs before and after the workout, and throughout if possible.

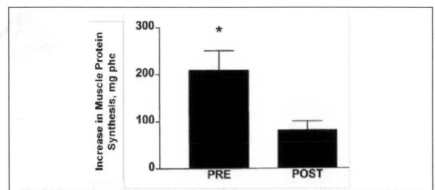

Figure 9.2. When EAAs were given before resistance exercise muscle protein synthesis was stimulated more than when given after exercise, but the EAAs given after exercise still caused a significant stimulation.

A high quality intact protein supplement can provide the EAAs necessary to stimulate muscle protein synthesis during or after resistance exercise. The intact protein also provides an abundant supply of NEAAs. However, the availability of the NEAAs is not at all limiting after a weight-lifting workout due to the accelerated breakdown of muscle protein (which releases both EAAs and NEAAs). Think of EAAs as the "active component" of protein. Also, depending on the protein, the delay in the time for digestion and absorption of the intact protein can dampen the EAA signal to the muscle. An EAA supplement can yield the greatest and most efficient response by rapidly providing the optimal profile of EAAs that combine with circulating NEAAs to effectively build more muscle and improve strength.

There is an interactive effect between resistance exercise and EAAs. Both stimulate muscle protein synthesis, and the combined effect is greater than either of their individual effects. You can consider it as if the resistance exercise "primes" the muscle to produce protein at an accelerated rate, but muscle protein synthesis is limited by the availability of EAAs in the fasted state. Ingested EAAs are rapidly consumed by the muscle, in part because the blood flow to muscle is increased by resistance exercise, and in part because the molecular mechanisms in the muscle cells that regulate the rate of synthesis are turned on. The net result is that the major gain in muscle mass that occurs after resistance exercise is due to the combined effects of the exercise and the increased availability of EAAs (**Figure 9.3**).

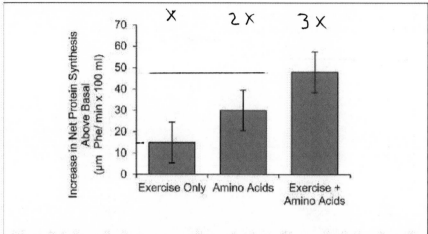

Figure 9.3. Interaction between exercise and amino acids on stimulation of muscle protein synthesis. The combined response is greater than the response to either one alone.

Different Approaches for Different Goals

The question that may occur to you is that the description of the interaction between resistance exercise and EAAs explains how you increase both strength and muscle mass, but what if your goal is to just increase muscle strength, without increasing mass? While my personal example of this goal was that of being a distance runner not wanting to add body weight, a more common example is women who want to get stronger without getting bigger. Strong is the new sexy, but this usually does not include "getting huge", which is a goal of a lot of men that are avid weight lifters.

The interesting thing is that the response of the muscle to resistance exercise and EAA supplementation depends on the workout. In the case of performing a few heavy lifts, the molecular signaling to enhance the synthetic response to the EAAs is amplified, such that the rate of synthesis will exceed the rate of breakdown when EAAs become available, and you will gain both strength and muscle mass. In contrast, when you do multiple lifts with a relatively small weight, muscle protein turnover will also be stimulated to a greater extent when EAAs are taken in conjunction with the workout, but there will be a closer balance between synthesis and breakdown and strength will increase without much change in muscle mass.

The non-protein component of an EAA supplement plays a role in determining the ultimate result of the exercise on strength and mass. If EAAs are taken with carbohydrate, the insulin response to the carbohydrate will enhance the EAA effect on muscle protein synthesis, suppress protein breakdown, and there will be a greater net gain of muscle protein. In addition, some of the carbohydrate will be stored in the muscle as glycogen, and water is attached to the glycogen in its storage form in muscle. As a result, the size of the muscle will increase even more than from the gain in net protein. However, because of the water and glycogen storage, muscle definition will be lessened. If you are trying to increase muscle mass and strength and not particularly worried about muscle definition, then you should take carbohydrate along with the EAAs before and after a workout.

If you are a body builder and want to get bigger but also want muscle definition, carbohydrate intake should be limited. This is true not only with regard to the EAA supplements, but in your basic diet as well. It is best to take only EAAs before and during the workout, and your regular diet should be composed of largely protein and fat. This will minimize the storage of glycogen and water in the muscle, both of which impair muscle definition. Also, the total caloric intake over the day will ultimately impact the increase in muscle mass.

If muscle strength and definition without much increase in mass is your specific goal, you should take EAAs by themselves before and after your workout. By performing a large number of repetitions with a relatively low weight, the net gain in muscle protein will be less than when you do a few lifts with heavy weights. It may be inevitable that you gain some muscle mass along with your gains in strength, even if you do multiple repetitions, but if you take the EAAs without carbohydrates before and after your workouts, the major impact will be on strength. You will also lose some fat for reasons discussed in the chapter on energy metabolism, with the result that your muscle definition will also increase.

Essentials

- "Substrate metabolism" in exercise refers to the fuels used to sustain activity. For most recreational activities, the body uses a mix of carbohydrate and fat.
- Carbohydrate in the body is the glucose circulating in blood and glycogen (glucose molecules linked together) stored in liver and muscle.
- Fat is stored as triglyceride (3 fatty acids linked together) and circulates as free fatty acids.
- Muscle protein is broken down during aerobic exercise. Energy can be derived from oxidation of released leucine.
- The "central fatigue hypothesis" refers to the increase in serotonin in the brain due to decreased leucine concentration in the blood. Serotonin is an inhibitory neurotransmitter that may amplify fatigue experienced during prolonged exercise.
- Consumption of EAAs following aerobic exercise can replace the amino acids broken down during exercise and enhance muscle recovery.
- Resistance exercise increases muscle mass and strength by increasing muscle protein turnover.
- Intact protein can increase muscle protein synthesis but it is not as efficient as EAAs since the NEAAs in the intact protein are not needed and the process of digestion and absorption can delay the peak increase in EAAs.
- EAAs can be thought of as the "active ingredient" of protein
- EAAs ingested before and after resistance exercise will be anabolic since the breakdown of muscle protein during exercise will be reversed and protein synthesis after exercise will be stimulated.
- Carbohydrate plus EAA/protein supplementation increases muscle mass but decreases muscle definition by promoting glycogen storage in the muscle.

Chapter 10. Aging

Loss of Muscle with Aging

As a scientist, I have had plenty of arguments in my career. Part of the scientific process is addressing challenges and defending your theories. One of the few things I have spoken about to audiences of scientists that has never been challenged is that we lose muscle mass and strength as we get older. I have never had someone shout from the audience "Hey, that's not right; I'm getting stronger as I get older". So, we can all agree that we lose muscle as we age. In about 30% of people, the loss of muscle becomes severe. The state of severe depletion of muscle mass with aging is called *sarcopenia*. Once someone suffers from sarcopenia, the functions of daily living are severely affected. Even if an individual has not lost enough muscle to be classified as sarcopenic, adverse health consequences can result from even a modest loss of muscle.

Consequences of Loss of Muscle Mass and Strength with Aging

Despite the widespread recognition that muscle mass and strength are lost with aging, the physiological significance of this loss is underappreciated. It is well recognized that you can't run as fast or hit the golf ball as far as you get older. If the loss of muscle strength becomes severe, basic activities of daily living can be affected, with significant adverse effects on quality of life. Perhaps even more importantly, loss of muscle mass and strength has much broader health implications. Recent research has made clear that significant loss of muscle mass and/or strength will increase your risk of cardiovascular events and decrease survival from various diseases including cancer and chronic obstructive lung disease. Also, recovery from major surgery is impaired and bone health suffers. These health issues are related to muscle mass. The reason that muscle is at the core of all these health conditions is due to muscle's role as the reservoir for amino acids (Chapter 2). This means that amino acids from muscle are mobilized when other tissues and organs need an increased supply of amino acids for all sorts of stresses; to battle infection, for wound repair, vascular control, metabolic balance, and more. Muscle also plays a role in maintaining a healthy energy balance.

A little background on the changes in muscle protein metabolism that occur with aging will help you understand why the EAASE program works so effectively and is so important for older individuals.

The Loss of Muscle Begins Before You Realize It

Quite often, people don't recognize that they have lost muscle mass and function until they are 70 years old or older. This oversight is particularly the case with people who don't participate in any organized recreational activities. They don't experience a quantitative feedback on performance. The reason that it is not easy to recognize the problems caused by the loss of muscle mass and function is because of what we call a "threshold effect".

The loss of muscle starts in some as early as age 30 and by age 50, almost everyone is starting to lose a significant amount of muscle. However, you may not notice this because your body weight doesn't change or may even go up (due to increased fat), and you can still comfortably perform the activities of daily living. As the loss of muscle progresses, basic function may still be maintained. Most commonly, this will be the case until there is (an inevitable) health set-back. The loss of muscle occurs even faster when there is serious illness, injury or surgery. When the normal age-related rate of muscle loss is coupled with the accelerated loss that occurs in response to a health crisis, function may all of a sudden be affected to the point where you notice a problem; the "threshold" has been reached.

The key aspect of the EAASE program with respect to exercise in older individuals is that it is much easier to maintain muscle mass than to regain it once lost. One of the reasons for this is that after you have lost a significant amount of function, you are limited in the amount of exercise you are able to perform. Secondly, since the muscle has been depleted, there are metabolic changes that make it less receptive to the beneficial effects of EAAs.

The bottom line is to try to maintain your muscle mass and function before you lose it. When you turn 50, it is time to get serious about maintaining your muscle (**Figure 10.1**).

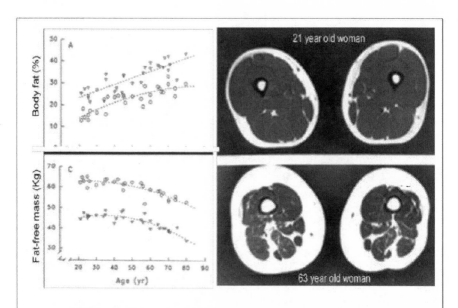

Figure 10.1. As we age, we gain fat and lose fat-free mass (i.e., muscle). The loss of muscle shown in the cross-sectional images on the right are vivid examples of how fat replaces muscle with aging.

140

Anabolic Resistance

The metabolic basis for the loss of muscle is that, over time, the rate of muscle protein breakdown exceeds the rate of synthesis. Interestingly, in the post-absorptive state (between meals), the rates of synthesis and breakdown do not change with aging. In contrast, there is a diminished increase in protein synthesis when dietary protein is consumed. Thus, normal protein nutrition is not as effective in elderly as in younger people. This dampened response is termed *anabolic resistance* and it is the principle reason why you lose muscle as you age. The nature of anabolic resistance is shown graphically in **Figure 10.2.** The same amount of EAAs in the profile found in whey protein elicits twice the stimulation of muscle protein synthesis in young individuals than older, healthy individuals

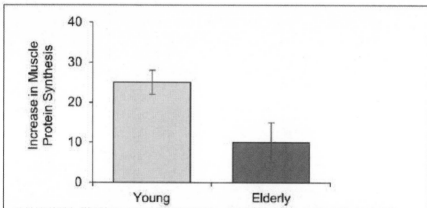

Figure 10.2. Anabolic resistance in aging. Muscle protein synthesis increases twice as much in young as compared to elderly subjects when each consume the same amount (7 g) of EAAs in the profile of the EAAs in whey protein. Free EAAs are fully absorbed, so the deficit in the response is due to a lack of responsiveness of the muscle (i.e., anabolic resistance).

If you recall from the overview of muscle, there is a specific control over muscle protein synthesis that involves a molecule called mTOR. mTOR acts as the "starter" in getting muscle building started. With aging, mTOR is less responsive to cues like amino acids and it takes more of the amino acid signal to get things going. This loss of sensitivity is the metabolic basis for anabolic resistance in aging.

Hormonal Changes with Aging

Women

Middle age in women is marked in part by menopause, which occurs around the age of 50. Many changes occur with menopause including the end of menstruation. Physiologically, the most important aspect of menopause is probably the reduction in secretion of female hormones from the ovaries. Most notably, estrogen secretion is reduced, but the secretion of other hormones is also reduced. Decreased secretion of estrogen after menopause contributes to deterioration in bone health. A number of other responses also occur after menopause, some of which are due to the effect of the lack of estrogen, some as a response to aging, and others that arise from a combination of these two factors.

Hormone replacement therapy (HRT) with estrogen and progestin has been used to counter the symptoms of menopause. While the prescription of HRT used to be common, side effects and complications like blood clotting and stroke have reduced the long-term use of HRT. Other medications may be prescribed for a more targeted therapy of specific symptoms of menopause.

Men

The predominant hormonal response to aging in men is reduced secretion of the hormone testosterone from the testes. Testosterone is the primary anabolic hormone in men. It promotes the gain of new muscle protein, and has other effects as well. Sexual function in older men is directly affected by a reduction in testosterone. Replacement therapy with testosterone is popular, although therapy is limited by the fact that testosterone cannot be given as a pill. Patches are commonly used to increase the testosterone level, but the amount of the hormone that can be delivered by this route is limited and insufficient to affect muscle. As a result, only some aspects of testosterone action can be restored by the use of testosterone patches. Most notably, sexual function, which includes both the level of interest in sex as well as the ability to do something about that interest, is improved when testosterone is given in a patch format. Testosterone must be injected, usually once per week or once every other week, to increase the concentration of testosterone enough to have an anabolic effect on muscle.

The use of testosterone replacement therapy is controversial because of worry that the growth of any existent prostate cancer may be stimulated by testosterone therapy. This fear arises from the fact that the first line of action in the treatment of prostate cancer is often giving a drug that blocks the action of testosterone on the prostate. Since this therapy can be effective, it gives reason for caution with the use of testosterone therapy.

Other Hormonal Responses to Aging

Insulin plays a crucial role in regulating the blood glucose level, and the development of diabetes is directly related to the loss of normal insulin action (*insulin resistance*). Insulin is also an anabolic hormone. Insulin stimulates muscle protein synthesis and inhibits muscle protein breakdown. Aging is accompanied by a decrease in the function of insulin. About 60% of people 65 years of age or older have some degree of insulin resistance. This condition can affect the way in which the body handles fuel, including carbohydrate and protein and may also contribute to loss of muscle mass.

Growth hormone is highly anabolic in growing children. Children who are deficient in growth hormone do not grow normally, and replacement of the hormone restores a normal growth rate. Growth hormone is greatly reduced with aging. Because of the effectiveness of growth hormone therapy in children with growth hormone deficiencies, growth hormone therapy is popular with older people. However, there is no evidence of a beneficial effect of growth hormone therapy in older people. It is not surprising that as you age, you lose responsiveness to growth hormone, since older people have stopped growing many years earlier. Growth hormone therapy can be associated with adverse responses, including an increase in insulin resistance. It is possible to stimulate growth hormone in older people with a supplement of lysine and arginine, but there is no evidence that this provides a beneficial response.

EAASE and Hormonal Therapy

Hormonal therapy is not part of the EAASE program. It is my personal belief that changes in hormonal secretion are a natural part of aging, and that unanticipated adverse responses to hormonal therapy are significant. Two of the underlying principles of the EAASE program is that the program is without risk of adverse response, and does not require physician supervision. Of course, before making changes in your diet or exercise level, you might want to discuss these changes with your physician at the outset. Introduction of hormonal therapy would require modifying both of those principles.

Although hormonal therapy is not part of the EAASE program, remember that the acronym stands for Essential Amino Acid Solutions for *Everyone*, and this includes older individuals already receiving hormonal therapy. Consider the situation of treatment with testosterone. Testosterone is similar to resistance exercise in that it primes the muscle to increase its rate of synthesis. It needs building blocks (i.e., dietary EAAs) to actually produce new protein. Since the EAASE program is based on supplying an adequate amount of EAAs through both the regular diet and EAA supplementation, following the EAASE program will amplify any beneficial effects of testosterone on muscle protein synthesis.

The EAASE program can also help with the problem of insulin resistance so common in older people. One of the characteristics of insulin resistance with aging is that fat accumulates in the liver and limits insulin action as a result. Older individuals have, on average, twice the fat in their livers than when they were under 30 years of age. EAA supplements reduce liver fat in elderly to the same degree as the most effective medication, and with none of the adverse effects of the medicine (Chapter 5). As a result, insulin sensitivity is improved. The exercise component of the EAASE program will also improve insulin sensitivity.

Dietary Protein Intake in the Elderly

Many of the consequences of suboptimal EAA intake become functionally evident with advancing age. Ideally, we want to curb these consequences before they are established. However, it is not too late to do something about loss of muscle mass and function even when someone reaches 65 or more years of age. Almost ironically, the usual dietary EAA intake tends to fall in older individuals, just when it would really make a positive impact on their lives to *increase* EAA intake. In America, 30% of people over the age of 65 fail to eat the minimal daily recommended intake of protein. Furthermore, the quality of the dietary protein also decreases, meaning that EAA intake is greatly reduced in many older people. Most prominently, meat intake decreases. This may occur for a variety of reasons, including high cost for people living on a fixed income, issues related to food preparation, problems chewing, digestive limitations, and changes in taste preferences. Unfortunately, people may also be reacting to advice to decrease their meat intake to benefit their health. Any or all of these factors may lead to an inadequate intake of high quality protein in meat.

Dietary supplementation has been marketed and used as therapy in older individuals, mostly with protein-enhanced beverages. The general idea is to provide some high-quality protein like whey protein to increase the EAA content of the diet since the typical diet is lacking in protein. However, intact protein supplements have not proven to be consistently helpful in all older individuals. The problem, as referred to above, is anabolic resistance. The normal action of dietary protein to stimulate muscle protein synthesis is diminished in the elderly. Consequently, even if enough supplemental protein is provided to bring the total EAA intake level up to an optimal level, loss of muscle mass and function will not be reversed.

Anabolic Resistance and the Optimal EAA Profile

One major advantage of free EAA formulations is that the profile of the EAAs can be precisely adjusted to be optimal for specific circumstances. In the case of the anabolic resistance of muscle protein that occurs with aging, the profile of EAAs in even a high quality protein is ineffective. My laboratory has done years of research to determine the optimal profile of EAAs to maximally stimulate muscle protein synthesis in the circumstance of anabolic resistance.

One of the key aspects of anabolic resistance is trouble getting the motor started. The starter for the motor in this case is the initiation factor we discussed before, mTOR. The EAA leucine is one of the most important regulators of mTOR activity. If the proportion of leucine in a mixture of EAAs is increased, the formulation of EAAs can effectively activate mTOR in aging muscle. However, leucine alone is not enough. I have previously referred to leucine as the quarterback of a football team. It may be the most important player, but you need all of the EAAs in the proper proportion to produce new protein.

When you consume a large amount of the EAA leucine, you increase the rate at which leucine gets broken down since the body is designed to maintain steady levels of EAAs. Coincidentally, the breakdown of all the BCAAs (leucine, valine, and isoleucine) is increased because the same enzyme works on all three BCAA. Consequently, the proportions of valine and isoleucine in the EAA formulation must also be increased to avoid decreases in their availability.

Lysine is another EAA with distinct characteristics. In the case of lysine, it is not transported into muscle as readily as other EAAs. Consequently, the optimal profile of EAAs to maximally stimulate "anabolic resistant" muscle includes proportionately more lysine than is reflected in the composition of muscle protein. So even though it may seem logical to provide EAAs for a muscle-building supplement in a profile similar to the makeup of muscle,

148

adjustments can be made to boost the signal and improve delivery of amino acids to overcome "anabolic resistance".

The other five EAAs (phenylalanine, threonine, methionine, tryptophan, and histidine) also need to be included in a mixture of EAAs to maximally stimulate muscle protein synthesis. The proportionate contribution of these additional EAAs must be reduced below what occurs in muscle protein because of the necessity of including disproportionately high amounts of BCAAs and lysine.

We showed in studies that the response of net muscle protein synthesis was improved to where the elderly increased as much as the young when a mixture of EAAs meeting the criteria outlined above was provided **(Figure 10.3).** A mixture of EAAs with this profile was three times more effective in stimulating muscle protein synthesis in older individuals on a gram/gram basis than whey protein isolate, which is a very high quality protein by traditional means of assessment. We also used this formulation of EAAs to decrease the loss of muscle mass and strength that occurs with bed rest and recovery from hip replacement. The difference between the effectiveness of EAAs and intact protein cannot be made up just by consuming more of the intact protein, because the optimal profile of EAAs will never be achieved with intact protein. It is a matter of quality, not quantity.

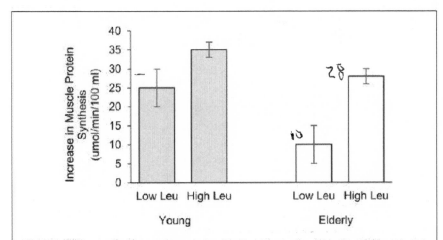

Figure 10.3. Anabolic resistance in older individuals (Figure 10.2) can be overcome by changing the profile of the EAA mixture to include 40% leucine. The response of net muscle protein synthesis to a high-leucine mixture of EAAs is the same in young and elderly.

150

- Loss of muscle mass and strength with aging has functional and health consequences.
- Loss of muscle becomes significant by age 50. This is the time to get serious about slowing the progression if you haven't already started.
- Hormonal changes with aging contribute to the loss of muscle. Hormone replacement therapies for both men and women may provide some benefit, but also have potential adverse effects.
- *Anabolic resistance* refers to the diminished effectiveness of intact protein in terms of stimulating muscle protein synthesis in older individuals.
- Consumption of high-quality dietary protein often decreases with aging.
- A specific EAA formulation can overcome anabolic resistance. The optimal formulation can be three times more effective in stimulating muscle protein synthesis than high-quality protein.

Chapter 11. Weight Loss

Health Risks of Obesity

Many of us feel that we would like to lose a few extra pounds, to look better and have our clothes fit better. But for too many Americans, those extra pounds keep adding up to the point that nearly 40% of Americans are classified as obese. Obese is defined as having a body mass index (BMI; weight (kg)/height^2 in meters) greater than 30. The cluster of health problems that accompany obesity including hypertension, unhealthy blood lipid profiles, and insulin resistance are referred to as the *metabolic syndrome*. More than 40% of individuals over the age of 60 suffer from the metabolic syndrome. The metabolic syndrome is the precursor for diabetes. In addition to increasing the likelihood of the metabolic syndrome, obesity causes physical disability due to the burden of carrying extra weight as well as joint pain resulting in part from increased inflammation. I talked earlier about preserving muscle mass and function as we age by starting early to minimize the loss of muscle rather than trying to restore muscle once it is lost. In the same fashion, taking action early to address extra pounds before obesity sets in is the most effective approach.

Healthy Eating Patterns and Obesity

We would all agree that eating a "healthy diet" is important to maintain a healthy body weight or to lose excess weight. It is much more difficult to get everyone to agree on what comprises a healthy diet. The 2015 Dietary Guidelines for Americans published by the USDA specifically states that a goal is to help people make decisions that help keep their weight under control and prevent chronic conditions like type 2 diabetes, hypertension, and heart disease. The emphasis in the updated version of guidelines is on "healthy eating patterns", recognizing that people don't typically eat a random collection of foods. Along with a healthy U.S. style eating pattern in the guidelines, there is a healthy Mediterranean style pattern and even a healthy vegetarian eating pattern. Specific recommendations promote fruits and vegetables, whole grains and healthy oils. Regarding protein, the guidelines suggest Americans should consume fat free and low fat dairy including milk, yogurt, cheese and/or fortified soy beverages. Also, "a variety of protein foods including seafood, lean meats, poultry, eggs, legumes (peas and beans), soy products, and nuts and seeds" should be included in the diet.

While variety may be "the spice of life", this move to promote the *variety* of proteins makes it increasingly difficult to obtain the optimal amount of EAAs within most people's caloric budget. In several sections of this book, I have stressed the physiological importance of the maintenance of a high rate of protein turnover, particularly in muscle. Dietary consumption of EAAs is the most effective thing you can do to maintain a high rate of muscle protein turnover. Animal proteins are the richest food source of EAAs, providing the most favorable amount and profile of EAAs in the fewest calories. Physiologically, we would expect that dietary recommendations to move away from consumption of animal proteins would favor the loss of lean mass and promote an increase in fat mass. This is exactly what has happened on a population basis in the United States.

In contrast to the USDA Dietary Guidelines for Americans, the EAASE program takes a physiological approach to the optimal dietary pattern. The heart of the EAASE program is maintaining the muscle mass and promoting a high rate of muscle protein turnover.

The Importance of Maintaining the Lean Mass during Weight Loss

Hopefully by now you are fully aware of how important it is to have "metabolically active muscle" to help you maintain energy balance. Obese younger individuals not only have increased fat mass, but muscle mass is usually increased as well. The increased muscle mass in younger, obese individuals stems from increased protein intake as part of an overall high-calorie diet. In contrast to the circumstance in young individuals, it is common in older individuals for debilitating loss of muscle mass to occur despite the presence of obesity. Severe loss of muscle mass and function in obesity occurs in about 30% of elderly individuals, and is termed *sarcopenic obesity*. Even in obese older individuals without sarcopenia *per se*, muscle mass and function is usually significantly lower than in younger counterparts. The combination of obesity and loss of muscle mass is the most debilitating combination possible for an older individual.

The reason that older people have lost muscle mass despite being obese can often be traced to lifestyle behaviors when they were younger. It is common for people who are inclined towards obesity to gain and lose weight multiple times throughout their lifetimes (yo-yo dieting). They may start out with increased muscle mass, but every time they lose weight, they lose fat and muscle, and then they regain weight almost entirely as fat. By the time they reach the age of 60, they have been through this cycle several times, with the result that they have depleted their muscle mass despite being obese. Thus, it is important to maintain muscle mass during weight loss even when you are still young.

Maintaining muscle mass during weight loss is important for physical function. While maintaining physical function is very important for us older folks, the role of muscle mass in maintaining energy balance may be more important for younger people, in a relative sense. Most young people have enough reserve so that they are more likely to be concerned about gaining unwanted weight than losing their physical function. The

155

processes of muscle protein synthesis and breakdown (i.e., muscle protein turnover) are going on continuously, and burning up calories in the process. The more muscle mass, the more energy expended to fuel muscle protein turnover, even in the basal state. Dietary EAAs stimulate muscle protein synthesis above the basal rate, and the more muscle mass you have, the greater the response of total protein synthesis. So, the more muscle that you have, the greater the increase in total caloric expenditure because of this accelerated muscle protein turnover. More calories burned translates to a better chance of maintaining a desirable weight. Maintaining a high rate of total muscle protein turnover is a cornerstone of the EAASE program for maintaining energy balance.

The Challenge of Maintaining Muscle Mass during Weight Loss

The nutritional challenge of maintaining muscle mass during weight loss is that in order to lose weight, it is necessary to cut back total caloric intake significantly. A diet providing about 1,200 kcal per day would be routine for caloric restriction weight loss. Even if dietary protein comprises 25% of total calories, with consumption of only 1,200 kcal, this would mean a total of only 300 kcal as protein, or 75 g. Protein intake of 75 g would provide the Recommended Dietary Intake (RDA) of protein (0.8 g body weight/kg/day) for someone weighing 93 kg, or 205 lbs. Keep in mind that this is the minimum amount of protein that can be eaten to maintain the lean body mass, and that minimal amount of protein is only adequate if total caloric requirements are met. This level of protein intake during caloric restriction weight loss is known to be inadequate to maintain muscle mass. Furthermore, a body weight of 205 lbs is probably at the low end of a weight for someone who would enter a caloric restriction weight loss program, particularly for a man.

At the risk of burdening you with too much math, here is another example to illustrate the challenge of obtaining adequate protein on a weight loss diet. Take a person who weighs 300 lbs and is beginning a diet of 1,200 kcal per day. This person would have to eat 36% of calories as protein to meet the minimal requirement of 0.8 g protein/kg/day, and that would be, in actuality, inadequate to maintain muscle mass because of the low caloric intake or energy availability. The RDA for protein is set in the context of having sufficient energy intake. In reality, at least 50% of calories would have to be eaten as protein to have a chance to preserve muscle mass during weight loss with a diet of 1,200 kcal/ day. In fact, high protein low-calorie diets have proven to preserve muscle mass better than traditional approaches. Unfortunately, a diet with such a high proportion of protein is difficult to sustain for a long period of time. Consequently, even with extremely high protein diets, it is difficult to preserve muscle mass during caloric restriction weight loss.

The challenge of increasing protein intake in a caloric restriction diet above what is normally eaten in an average diet in energy balance is illustrated in **Figure 11.1**.

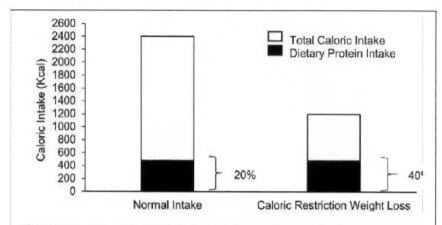

Figure 11.1. Example of the challenge of maintaining sufficient protein intake during caloric restriction weight loss. Assume that the normal caloric intake for energy balance is 2,400 kcal/day, 20% of which is dietary protein (left hand column). If the caloric intake is reduced to 1,200 kcal/day for weight loss, the same protein intake increases to 40 % of caloric intake (right hand column). This is above the upper limit of the AMDRs, but may nonetheless be inadequate to preserve muscle mass during weight loss because of the drop in caloric intake.

How Well Do High Protein Diets Work?

The theory supporting the benefit of a high protein diet for preserving muscle mass while losing weight is solid. The problem, as described above, is actually eating a "high protein" diet in the context of a reduced-calorie diet. Nonetheless, it is useful to examine the results of past studies that have used different amounts of protein in the diet.

Overall, research protocols testing the effectiveness of high protein weight loss diets find that most people can successfully lose weight with this approach. In many cases, these diets yield favorable changes in body composition as characterized by less loss of lean body mass compared to diets with low or standard protein intake. A recent extensive analysis of high protein diets analyzed the results of 46 different groups of subjects over the age of 50 that participated in caloric restriction weight loss programs. Half the groups of dieters were classified as "normal "and half as "high" protein intake. The break point was protein consumption equal to or greater than 1.0 gram protein/kg body weight /day, or 25% of caloric intake as protein. The range of protein intake was from 0.58-0.97 gram protein/kg body weight /day (15-22% of caloric intake) in the normal protein intake groups. The high protein intake groups ranged from1.01-1.57 g protein/kg body weight/day (25-40% of caloric intake). The BMIs ranged from 29.6 to 36.0, and the duration of diets ranged from 8 to 52 weeks.

The most important general finding was that the high protein groups retained more lean mass and lost more fat mass than the normal protein groups. Forty-seven percent of the normal protein groups lost more than 5 % of their lean body mass, while only 20 % of the high protein group lost a similar percentage of their lean body mass. Conversely, in the normal protein group, loss of fat mass constituted 57% of the total weight loss, while 78% of the total weight loss was fat mass in the high protein group. The same trend was seen when the absolute loss of lean mass was expressed in the units of kilograms. Importantly, none of the 46 groups of dieters maintained all of their lean body mass while undergoing caloric restriction weight loss.

The results of this detailed analysis of past research studies were predictable, based on the requirements for dietary protein to maintain a balance between protein synthesis and breakdown during caloric restriction weight loss. A diet containing less than 1.0 gram of protein/kg body weight /day is clearly deficient in protein and will result in significant loss of lean body mass. A higher intake of dietary protein not only better preserves muscle mass during weight loss, but also enhances the amount of fat loss. The practical problem is that even the highest protein intake tested out of all these studies that were reviewed (1.5 gram protein /kg body weight/day) is barely above the average daily intake under normal conditions. Given the relation between the amount of protein in the diet and the extent of preservation of lean body mass during weight loss, it could be expected that muscle could be completely preserved if the protein intake was increased to an even higher amount than 1.5 gram protein /kg body weight/day. Practically, that is difficult to accomplish with intact protein. For this reason, the EAASE program takes advantage of EAA supplementation of the diet to achieve an intake of EAAs in excess of what can possibly be consumed using only intact protein food sources.

The Composition of High-Protein Diets

In previous chapters, the importance of dietary protein was emphasized, particularly high quality protein with abundant essential amino acids (EAAs), in maintaining muscle protein mass and function. I also talked about enhanced energy expenditure due to dietary protein induced acceleration of protein turnover. Based on these physiological principles, "high-protein" diets have proven to be effective (as discussed above) and as a result have gained popularity and acceptance. There is a wide range of approaches within the general category of high protein diets. For the most part, these diets are all based on the intake of an abundant amount of high-quality protein. The major difference between these diets is the non-protein component of the diet.

Since there are only three macronutrients (protein, carbohydrate, and fat) or four if you consider alcohol, adjusting one component inevitably means altering one or all of the other components. Further, the amount of caloric restriction varies with different diets. In a diet containing a high proportion of protein, the amount of fat and/or carbohydrate also must change from the normal. In many cases the non-protein component of the diet may take center stage in the rationale of the diet, even if it is a high protein diet. It is possible that the benefits of a high-protein diet may be due at least in part to the reduction in one of the non-protein components of the diet. Nonetheless, it is important to realize that differences in the non-protein components of the diet notwithstanding, the crucial aspect of low calorie diets with regard to preservation of lean body mass is the amount and quality of protein.

There are several well-known high protein diets that recommend approximately 30% of calories as protein. These diets carve out their niche based mainly on the amount and source of carbohydrates and fat. I will discuss some of the most popular plans.

Popular High Protein Diets

There are a variety of diets that can be classified as high protein based on including at least 30% of caloric intake in the form of protein. From the above discussion, you should keep in mind that 30% of calories as protein may mean little or no increase in the actual amount of protein eaten as compared to the individual's normal diet. All of the diets are similar with regard to their recommendations for protein intake, reflecting the fact that there is a practical limit to the percent of the diet that can be comprised of protein, given the obligatory non-protein calories that are consumed along with the dietary protein with a high density of protein. Most of the high protein diets are further consistent in their recommendations to rely on animal sources of dietary proteins. This is necessary not only because of the recognized importance of the quality of the dietary protein, but from the practical standpoint that high protein density in protein food sources is essential if there is to be any flexibility in the remaining part of the diet.

The following are some of the most popular "high protein" diets.

The famous **Atkins** diet plan is an excellent example in which the non-protein component of the diet takes center stage, but in reality, benefits of the diets are likely due in large part to the high content of protein in the diet. The Atkins diet is predicated on the concept of minimizing carbohydrate in the diet in order to produce a state of ketosis. Ketosis refers to the production of chemicals called ketones that result when there is a high rate of fatty acid oxidation. The theory of the diet is that the ketones protect the skeletal muscle from degradation. The Atkins Diet website promotes that at least 70 grams of protein should be eaten, which would only be about 20% of caloric intake and therefore the diet does not qualify as high protein. In practice, however, the food choices in the Atkins diet will result in approximately 30% or more of caloric intake as protein. While the theory of the diet is based on the exclusion of carbohydrate rather than the amount of protein eaten, any beneficial effect might just as well be due to the high protein aspect of the diet as to the lack of carbohydrate.

The **Zone Diet** was proposed by Dr. Barry Sears based on the idea that the ideal ratio of macronutrient intake will reduce diet-induced inflammation and accelerate the loss of weight. The plan promotes a diet based on 40 % carbohydrate, 30% protein, and 30% fat. However, it is not clear if the diet really includes 30% as protein. Specifically, it is stated that lean proteins including egg whites, fish, poultry, lean beef, and low-fat dairy protein should comprise 1/3 of your plate, with carbohydrates in the form of colorful vegetables making up the other 2/3 of the plate along with a little fruit. High sugar fruits and starchy vegetables are not recommended. The remaining calories should come from the fat inherent in the protein foods and additional monounsaturated fat; for example, olive oil, avocados, or almonds. Omega-3 fatty acids are also emphasized to boost the anti-inflammatory benefits of the diet. The discrepancy is that 1/3 of your plate as foods such as fish, poultry, etc., will mean an actual protein intake of approximately 20% because of the non-protein components of the protein food sources.

The **South Beach Diet** is also considered a high-protein diet because it recommends that 30% of calories be eaten in the form of protein. As with other diets that could be considered high protein, the South Beach diet emphasizes the non-protein components of the diet. It takes the approach that a low glycemic index diet is crucial for weight management and metabolic health. Glycemic index is a system that ranks foods on a scale from 1 to 100 based on their effect on blood-sugar levels. Very much like the Zone diet, the basic diet is a balance of "good carbs", lean protein and healthy fats. "Bad carbs" are defined by the glycemic index and glycemic load to determine which carbs you should avoid. The South Beach Diet also promotes different kinds of dietary fats and encourages you to limit unhealthy fats, while eating more foods with healthier monounsaturated fats. The initial phase of the diet is almost carbohydrate free with the focus on lean protein such as seafood, skinless poultry, lean beef, and soy products. Ultimately, carbohydrates make up ~30% of calories mainly from fiber and whole grains, including fruits and vegetables as well as the carbohydrates found in low-fat dairy products.

The **Paleo Diet** or Paleolithic Diet is based on the idea that we should eat only foods presumed to be available to Paleolithic humans. This pattern is described to include 55% of daily calories from seafood and lean meat. This translates to about 30-35% of calories as protein when account is taken of the protein density of the recommended protein food sources. The remainder of the calories are divided evenly among fruits, vegetables, nuts and seeds. Restricted foods include dairy, most grains, and no added salt or sugar. Like all the other popular diets, this plan emphasizes avoiding processed and sugar sweetened foods.

It is interesting that, despite the unique "spin" for each of these diets, they all fundamentally fall into the category of balanced, nutrient dense dietary patterns that prescribe the upper range of the recommended level of dietary protein intake in terms of percent of calories consumed. In all cases, however, the amount of dietary protein is likely to be insufficient to preserve muscle mass during weight loss. The amount of protein in a low-calorie diet plan is limited by practical issues of protein density in naturally-occurring protein food sources. The caloric value of the non-protein components of dietary protein food sources may exceed the total amount of calories allowed by the diet. The consumption of EAAs as dietary supplements or incorporated into a food source, such as a meal replacement beverage, is likely the only way to achieve adequate EAA intake in the context of a calorically-restricted diet. FOR WEIGHT LOSS.

How High Should "High-Protein" Be?

The summary of the analysis of the impact of protein content of the diet on the nature of weight loss demonstrated conclusively that protein intake below 1.0 gram protein/kg body weight /day will result in a physiologically–significant loss of lean body mass. The analysis does not tell us the optimal amount of dietary protein. Keep in mind that although lean body mass was better preserved in those receiving a higher protein intake, none of the 46 groups entirely preserved their lean body mass. Based on the relationship between dietary protein intake and protein synthesis, it seems likely that at least 1.5 grams of protein/kg/day is required to reduce the loss of lean body mass to a minimal amount in most people. This would amount to about 40% of caloric intake as protein. Since we don't eat pure protein, that amount of protein intake could translate to as much as 80% or more of total caloric intake of the diet coming from protein foods.

The examples of the popular "high protein" diet plans described above makes clear that there is a practical limit to the amount of protein that can conveniently be included in a low-calorie diet. Unfortunately, this is not sufficient protein to entirely preserve muscle mass, particularly in older individuals.

The EAASE program includes consumption of supplemental dietary EAAs during caloric restriction weight loss in order to preserve muscle mass while losing weight. Dietary EAA supplements have no requisite non-protein component, and therefore have a minimal caloric value. Enough EAAs can be included in a low calorie diet to exceed what would be consumed in even a high-protein diet relying entirely on food sources. The fact that a proper formulation of EAAs is more effective in stimulating muscle protein synthesis than an intact protein is an added bonus.

Exercise During Weight Loss to Maintain Muscle Mass.

The best approach to maintaining lean body mass while losing fat mass is to combine exercise with a high protein caloric restriction diet. The principal benefit of exercise in weight loss is conventionally thought of in terms of increasing the caloric expenditure side of the energy balance equation. Indeed, it has been shown that when older individuals maintained a constant caloric intake and energy expenditure was increased 1,500 kcal per week by participation in a supervised exercise program of stationary cycling, they lost weight as predicted by the imbalance between energy expenditure and energy intake. Further, the loss was entirely as pounds from fat- lean body mass was conserved. From these results, it is clear that combining caloric restriction and aerobic exercise like stationary biking should work together to accelerate weight loss and preserve muscle mass.

While the logic of combining aerobic exercise and caloric restriction to preserve muscle mass during weight loss is sound, some research studies have reported that aerobic exercise does not preserve lean mass during caloric weight loss. Cumbersome and costly programs that combine supervised exercise training and dietary modification have often produced minimal alterations in body weight and physical function. While aerobic exercise is always beneficial in theory, not only in terms of energy balance but with regard to cardiovascular and metabolic health, enlisting in a costly or inconvenient exercise program that focuses on increasing your caloric expenditure through aerobic exercise may not be the most efficient way to lose weight or to maintain your muscle mass during dieting. The principle benefit of performing aerobic exercise such as cycling or walking while participating in a caloric restriction weight loss program is probably the cardiovascular and metabolic responses. Also, it helps you to establish a routine that you can carry out to maintain the health benefits of the weight loss after caloric restriction is completed. On the other hand, the amount of calories you will expend performing the aerobic exercise is unlikely to have a major impact on the amount of weight you lose. Losing weight requires caloric restriction.

One of the reasons why even supervised aerobic exercise can fail to make an impact on a weight loss program is that very overweight/obese individuals and many older people have a reduced aerobic exercise capacity. The amount of time that would need to be invested per day exercising to increase caloric expenditure enough to have a significant impact on weight loss is unrealistic. For example, it requires a trained athlete approximately 190 minutes of exercise at 50% peak oxygen consumption to burn the number of calories equivalent to one pound of fat. Peak oxygen consumption is a measure of a person's maximal capacity to perform aerobic exercise. Percentages of the "max" are used to describe the level of effort put forth in an activity. An older person exercising at the same percent of peak oxygen consumption requires 885 minutes to burn the same number of calories. This example reflects that 50% of a very low number (i.e., the peak oxygen consumption for an older, obese individual) translates to a very low amount of calories burned. In addition to the issue of the decline in aerobic fitness with aging and obesity, obese elderly have a high incidence of joint pain that significantly impairs their ability to exercise. It is true that studies have shown benefits of aerobic exercise during caloric restriction weight loss diets, but these studies have carefully screened potential subjects to ensure that they can comply with the protocol. The reality is that for obese and older people in particular, the contribution of aerobic exercise towards weight loss efforts is limited.

Given the limited effectiveness of aerobic exercise in older individuals in terms of weight loss, it may be quite surprising that resistance exercise can have a very positive impact on the outcome of a weight loss program. This is because resistance exercise amplifies the efficiency of the stimulation of muscle protein synthesis by dietary protein. The interaction between resistance exercise and dietary protein results in two beneficial outcomes. Stimulation of muscle protein synthesis is the metabolic basis for retention of muscle mass during weight loss. Also, the stimulation of muscle protein turnover requires increased energy expenditure.

The stimulation of muscle protein synthesis lasts for at least 48 hours after completion of resistance exercise. Thus, resistance exercise increases the amount of muscle protein that is using energy in the process of protein turnover, and the rate of muscle protein turnover is increased as well.

Since the central argument against relying heavily on aerobic exercise in a weight loss program for older obese individuals relates to the difficulty of performing the exercise, it would seem like the same would apply to resistance exercise. However, even physically disabled older individuals are capable of performing enough resistance exercise to benefit. In a study of nursing home residents over the age of 90 who were all confined to wheel chairs, a resistance exercise program improved their physical capability to the point that all were able to get out of their wheel chairs and walk and perform other activities of daily living. Even if you are somewhat disabled, it is possible that you could benefit from resistance exercise during weight loss.

The reason resistance exercise is effective in the context of weight loss, even in individuals with severe physical limitations, is that the amount of weight lifted that is required to stimulate muscle protein synthesis is very moderate, particularly when coupled with aggressive protein intake. Further, it has been shown that equal gains in strength result from multiple repetitions of very light weight as can be achieved with fewer repetitions of heavier weights. For older, obese individuals in weight reduction programs, incorporating resistance exercise using light weights and multiple repetitions will yield positive results in terms of both preservation of muscle mass and function and loss of fat mass.

The above discussion is not meant to imply that there is no benefit to aerobic exercise during a weight loss program. Cardiovascular and metabolic benefits result from aerobic exercise, even in the absence of weight loss, and caloric expenditure can be increased to some extent. Rather, we are emphasizing the importance of maintaining muscle protein turnover during weight loss, and the underappreciated fact that this may be most readily accomplished with resistance exercise.

The Need for an Alternative Approach to Muscle Preservation during Caloric Restriction Weight Loss

More often than not, weight loss diets have focused on the total amount of weight loss, rather than the nature of the weight loss (i.e., muscle mass vs fat mass). Hopefully, I have emphasized the importance of preserving muscle mass during weight loss. The most efficient way to accomplish this goal is to incorporate EAAs into the diet. EAAs can be taken either as dietary supplements or the EAAs can be incorporated into a meal replacement beverage. We recently conducted a study of caloric restriction weight loss in older individuals using a meal replacement beverage that included an EAA formulation optimized to promote muscle protein turnover. Those individuals who received the EAAs lost more fat with less muscle loss than those using a traditional meal replacement product.

EAAs can help you to overcome the limitations of weight loss diets, even high-protein weight loss diets, in terms of preserving muscle mass. Both protein-based and EAA-supplemented approaches are predicated on the maintenance of muscle mass through stimulation of muscle protein synthesis. Since the EAAs are approximately three-fold more efficient in stimulating muscle protein synthesis than high quality protein, the diet can rely on a more reasonable and calorically efficient amount of EAAs as opposed to intact protein. If a meal substitute is being used, it is necessary that some NEAAS also be included since a diet relying entirely on EAAs would eventually deplete the NEAAs. The proper balance can easily be achieved by the addition of a small amount of intact protein.

EAAs and Energy Balance

One of the challenges of weight loss is that as your body adapts to a low caloric intake, your metabolic rate slows down. So, assuming you are in energy balance when you start the weight loss program and you are expending and eating about 2,400 kcal per day, when the caloric intake is reduced from 2,400 kcal to 1,200 per day, you will initially have an energy imbalance of approximately 1,200 kcal per day. Since it takes an energy imbalance of about 3,500 kcal to lose one pound of fat, you will start losing weight at the rate of about 1 pound of fat every 3 days, presuming all weight loss is fat. (More about the energetics of losing muscles as compared to fat is discussed below). However, after a week or so, your metabolic rate will slow as your body adapts to the reduced calorie intake. It may slow about 10-15%, meaning that instead of burning 2,400kcal per day, you are burning about 2,100kcal per day. If you continue with the 1,200 kcal/day diet, you will now take four days to lose the same pound of fat that took you three days to lose earlier in the program. Not a big difference, but enough to get discouraged by what seems to be a plateauing in your progress. EAAs will help you out with this problem of reduced energy expenditure with a reduced-calorie diet in two ways: diet-induced thermogenesis and increased basal rate of protein synthesis.

Diet-Induced Thermogenesis

The metabolic rate goes up about 10% for a couple of hours after the meal when you eat dietary protein. The amount of increase depends on how much protein you eat with the meal. This response has been studied for many years and is called diet-induced thermogenesis. Diet-induced thermogenesis refers to energy lost as heat after you eat protein. Diet induced thermogenesis only applies to dietary protein, as neither dietary carbohydrate nor fat have much effect on the metabolic rate. In the case of a meal containing dietary protein, the metabolic rate increases because energy is used to digest the protein and absorb

170

the resulting amino acids. In addition, a meal containing dietary protein increases the metabolic rate by stimulating the rate of protein synthesis in the body, particularly in muscle, since the process of synthesis requires energy (Chapter 3).

The stimulation of metabolic rate resulting from diet-induced thermogenesis of dietary protein means that the functional calories ingested in the form of protein are actually less than calculated by the traditional approach. Calories are classically determined by combusting the food source in a device that measures the energy released. In the case of protein, 4 kcal/g of protein are normally released by combustion, so the caloric-equivalency of protein is traditionally considered to be 4 kcal/g. In other words, you can calculate how many protein calories there are in a meal by multiplying the grams of protein by 4 kcal/gm. However, since the digestion of protein increases metabolic rate approximately 10%, the net caloric intake from the protein component of the meal is actually 10% less than determined by the traditional approach. This means that on a 1,200 kcal/ day diet, if 35% of the diet is protein, then you will functionally be consuming only 1,158 kcal. This would translate to about an additional pound of fat lost every 83 days as compared to the rate of loss without the diet-induced thermogenesis. This is one of the benefits of a high-protein diet for weight loss although you can see from the math that this aspect of protein nutrition alone is insufficient to rely on as an important aspect of weight management.

A diet based on EAAs will have a greater diet-induced thermogenesis than protein (**Figure 11.2**). Even though the energy cost of the digestion of EAAs may be lower than intact protein, on a gram/gram basis, EAAs will stimulate protein synthesis about 3 times more than intact protein. If you consume 5 doses (15 g each) per day of EAAs, each dose will maximally stimulate protein synthesis. As a result, the increase in metabolic rate due to diet-induced thermogenesis will be elevated above the basal rate for at least 10 hours per day. Furthermore, the magnitude of the stimulation of protein synthesis will be greater when EAAs are ingested as opposed to intact protein. This response translates to an overall increase in metabolic rate of about 30% of the amount of calories consumed as EAAs. So, if you consume 5 x 15 g doses of EAAs per day, you would be consuming 300 kcal by traditional measurement of caloric value, but in reality, the true caloric value of the EAAs would be approximately 210 kcal/day. If you consider that 90 kcal/day difference in the context of a total daily intake of 1,200 kcal/day, a net of only about 1,110 kcal/day would be consumed. This means that the diet-induced thermogenesis resulting from consumption of EAAs would translate to losing an extra pound of fat every 39 days as compared to a diet based on dietary protein, even when as much as 35% of calories are given as dietary protein.

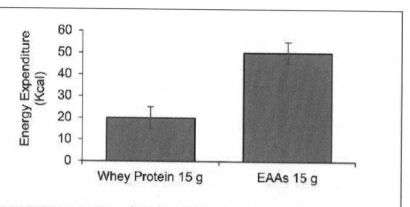

Figure 11.2. Consumption of dietary protein increases metabolic rate for about two hours after a meal. This is called diet-induced thermogenesis. Diet-induced thermogenesis was more than twice as much when the same amount of EAAs were given, due to the greater stimulation of protein synthesis. The difference between the diet-induced thermogenesis from EAAs vs protein translates to about 4 lbs more fat loss per year with the EAAs.

The importance of the difference between the protein-based approach to weight loss and the EAA-based approach can be appreciated if an entire 16 week weight loss protocol is considered. Thus, over 16 weeks the metabolic response to the high protein diet will translate to a little over a pound of fat loss, whereas the metabolic response to the EAA-based approach will translate to approximately 3 pounds of fat loss. . The diet-induced thermogenesis works for you in this way regardless of whether you are trying to lose weight or to maintain your hard-earned new weight.

The basal metabolic rate refers to the rate of energy production when you are inactive and not absorbing food. The best time to determine your basal metabolic rate is when you are sleeping. The same basic metabolic functions that determine the basal rate of energy expenditure also proceed when you are active. During the day, your total metabolic expenditure is the sum of your basal rate (which occurs continuously) and a factor for your level of activity. It is the basal metabolic rate that slows down as you adapt to a low calorie diet. When your basal metabolic rate slows, it works against you when you are trying to lose weight.

Your metabolic rate slows when you are losing weight because protein synthesis slows, thereby requiring less energy. This decrease in metabolic rate is an adaptive response to low energy intake. However, it is especially important when you are trying to lose weight to maintain your rate of protein synthesis in order to maximize your energy expenditure. Numerous examples in this book show how protein synthesis, particularly in muscle, is stimulated in response to EAA consumption. The stimulation of muscle protein synthesis is important during weight loss to preserve muscle mass. Also, the increase in protein synthesis after a meal is the basis of the diet-induced thermogenesis discussed above. The important information in this section is that EAA consumption also increases the basal rate of muscle protein synthesis, thereby increasing the basal metabolic rate (**Figure 11.3**).

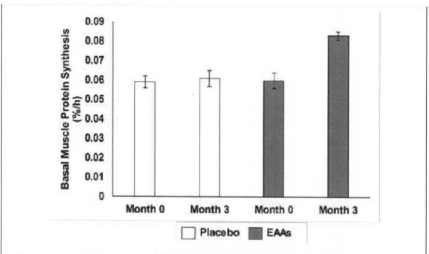

Figure 11.3. Three months of EAA supplementation caused an increase in the basal rate of muscle protein synthesis in older individuals while the placebo caused no change.

By basing the diet for the EAASE program for weight loss primarily on EAAs rather than protein, not only is muscle preserved, but the fall in metabolic rate that usually occurs when dieting is prevented. The maintenance of the normal rate of energy expenditure throughout dieting is due to the combined effects of diet-induced thermogenesis and the stimulation of the basal rate of protein synthesis. The net result is the preferential loss of fat mass relative to muscle, and a more rapid loss of fat.

The Energetics of Losing Fat and Preserving Muscle

The importance of losing fat and preserving muscle mass during weight loss is a fundamental principle of the EAASE program. The physiological and metabolic benefits of weight loss are due entirely to the loss of fat. Improvement in physical function, insulin sensitivity and blood lipids are directly related to the decrease of fat mass relative to muscle mass. Muscle is responsible for improved physical function after the loss of fat, as well as the clearance of glucose from the blood. Loss of fat is the primary reason that blood lipid profiles are improved with weight loss. Aesthetically, you will look better if you lose fat as opposed to muscle because muscle is denser and therefore occupies less volume than a calorically-equivalent amount of fat. Also, improving the ratio of fat/muscle will help significantly in the maintenance of weight loss after the period of dieting.

The EAASE program for weight loss involves the use of EAA-based meal replacements to preserve muscle mass during weight loss by maximally stimulating muscle protein synthesis. The maximal stimulation of muscle protein synthesis several times per day preserves muscle mass and also increases the resting metabolic rate as well as the dietary–induced thermogenesis.

The question arises as to why such an extensive reliance on EAAs to maximally stimulate muscle protein synthesis several times per day is necessary to preserve muscle mass during weight loss. The answer to that question is that energetics of fat and muscle tissue work against the preservation of muscle during weight loss.

Muscle is much denser than fat tissue due to the greater protein and water content of muscle. As a result, approximately 700 kcals of energy are stored in one pound of muscle, while approximately 3,500 kcals of energy are stored in a pound of fat. Expressed differently, if all other things are equal, it requires a caloric deficit of 3,500 kcal to lose a pound of fat, while it requires an energy deficit of only 700 kcal to lose a pound of muscle.

A numerical example will help to clarify the significance of the different amounts of energy stored in muscle and fat. Consider the case of a 3,500 kcal deficit in energy balance. This means that energy expenditure exceeds caloric intake by 3,500 kcal. This would probably take 3-4 days of caloric restriction weight loss. If 100% of the weight loss was fat, 1 pound of fat would be lost because 3,500 kcal of energy are stored in one pound of fat. Alternatively, if 100% of weight loss was muscle, then 5 pounds of muscle would be lost, because only 700 kcal of energy is stored in one pound of muscle, and 5 times 700 kcal would equal the 3,500 kcal energy deficit. The usual nature of weight loss without adequate dietary EAAs/ protein and without exercise is a mixture of fat and muscle. In this case, a 3,500 kcal deficit will produce a weight loss between 1 and 5 pounds.

Many weight- loss programs capitalize on the fact that it is easier to lose a pound of muscle than a pound of fat by utilizing a diet that initially fosters extensive loss of muscle and water. The early rapid weight loss is encouraging to the client and inspires devotion to the program, even though those early weight gains slow down considerably. Further, the expected long-term benefits of the weight loss are usually not obtained.

The beneficial effects of dietary EAAs on energy balance work to offset the differences in stored energy in fat and muscle. Nonetheless, it is possible that a weight loss program utilizing an EAA- based meal replacement will not induce more rapid weight loss than an approach that causes a rapid depletion of muscle mass and loss of body water. While the appeal of rapid initial weight loss on a diet is undeniable, it should take a back seat in importance to the preservation of muscle during weight loss. It is therefore important that the inspiration for weight loss is a desire to achieve the long-term benefits of preserving muscle mass during weight loss.

The EAASE program for weight loss targets the loss of fat mass and the complete preservation of muscle mass. The long-term results of weight loss with the EAASE program will be better maintenance of the new weight, and long-lasting improvements in health outcomes and physical function.

Essentials

- Obesity is a major health crisis in the United States. Traditional dietary guidelines have not slowed the rate of increase in obesity. The latest guidelines promote eating a variety of proteins which may dilute the overall quality of protein eaten and compromise EAA intake.
- Caloric restriction weight loss usually involves loss of both muscle and fat, but preservation of muscle mass during weight loss is important.
- Preserving muscle mass during weight loss is difficult with traditional dietary approaches because the required percentage of caloric intake as protein is often impractical.
- Both resistance and aerobic exercise can help to preserve muscle mass during caloric restriction weight loss, but exercise alone is generally ineffective for losing weight. Caloric restriction is necessary to lose weight.
- Diets with higher amounts of protein preserve lean body mass better during weight loss than those with less protein.
- All "high protein diets" for weight loss have about the same amount of protein (about 30% of caloric intake)
- Relying on EAAs as a central dietary component during caloric restriction weight loss can preserve muscle and accelerate fat loss by stimulating the basal rate of muscle protein synthesis.
- Diet-induced thermogenesis as well as increasing the basal rate of muscle protein turnover can help to preserve muscle and accelerate fat loss by increasing the metabolic rate for several hours after EAA intake.

[handwritten margin note: NOT TRUE IF FUNG OBESITY CODE IS CORRECT]

178

Chapter 12. Response to Serious Illness and Disease, Injury, or Surgery

One of the cornerstones of the EAASE program is that it relies on natural nutritional components with no known side effects and can be undertaken without medical supervision. It may seem odd to include a chapter in this book addressing conditions that will surely involve medical care at some point. Indeed, I am not intending that the EAASE program would substitute for or conflict with direct care of a physician. However, it is unfortunately true that at some point in our lives, many of us have to deal with major surgery, serious illness such as pneumonia, or chronic disease such as kidney disease. There may be a phase in your treatment when nutritional therapy is part of your care, but more commonly you will be on your own for taking care of your nutritional needs. This point is particularly true for recovery from orthopedic surgery that many of us need as we age, but is also the case in recovery from any type of serious illness, ranging from a bad case of the flu to something so serious that you end up in intensive care. Even with the recognized importance of the role of nutrition in cancer recovery, detailed nutritional advice is rarely provided in standard treatment programs. Many of the concepts of the EAASE program are derived from my 30 years of experience in the nutritional and metabolic care of patients with severe burn injury and other forms of critical illness. The EAASE program is based on solid nutritional and metabolic principles and is consistent with nutritional guidelines provided by all national and international committees involved with the care of seriously ill patients.

The Catabolic State, or Stress Response

In a previous chapter, we focused on the adverse effects of muscle loss with aging on physical function and long-term health outcomes. The consequences of muscle loss as a result of serious injury or illness can be even more severe and more immediate. Muscle mass in critical illness can be a direct contributor to survival, as well as to the speed and extent of recovery. In contrast to the case in aging, where the loss of muscle mass is slow and occurs over years, serious illness or injury causes muscle loss at a rate so fast that consequences can be evident in a matter of days or weeks.

The rate of muscle loss with aging is slow enough that it has been difficult to determine the underlying metabolic basis for the loss. Very minor changes in protein synthesis and breakdown can result in significant changes in muscle mass when extended out over years, as is the case in aging. In contrast, serious illness, injury or surgery cause dramatic losses in muscle mass. The rapid loss of muscle is called a catabolic state, which is part of an overall response that can be considered a physiological *stress response*. There are common aspects of the stress response, regardless of the underlying cause (i.e., cancer, injury, surgery, etc.). The stress response not only involves the loss of muscle at a rate that is much faster than would occur in the absence of food intake (the catabolic state), but also includes loss of appetite as well as metabolic changes such as a reduced sensitivity to the action of the hormone insulin. The loss of appetite results in decreased nutritional intake at a time when demand for dietary nutrients, particularly protein, is increased. Interestingly, regardless of the clinical condition that causes the stress response, changes in muscle protein metabolism are basically the same. Therefore, I will discuss the stress response in a general context.

Muscle Protein Metabolism in the Stress Response

The rapid loss of muscle protein reflects an imbalance between the rates of protein synthesis and breakdown. This imbalance in the stress response is driven by a large increase in the rate of muscle protein breakdown (**Figure 12.1**). It is not unusual for the rate of protein breakdown to be increased by more than three fold. The flood of EAAs into the muscle cells resulting from the rapid rate of protein breakdown stimulates muscle protein synthesis. Even under these conditions, the message sent by the availability of EAAs is to build muscle. However, the increased synthesis is not enough to balance the increase in breakdown. The net result is a large increase in the loss of muscle protein in the post-absorptive state.

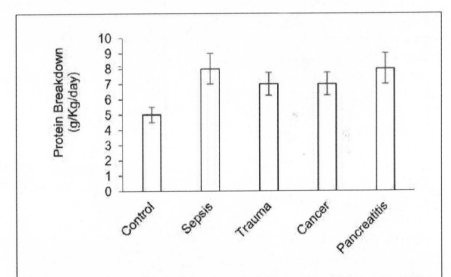

Figure 12.1. Protein breakdown is accelerated in any form of serious or critical illness or injury. This leads to a rapid loss of muscle mass that impairs recovery. The loss of muscle mass is a central part of the stress response. The basic aspects of the stress response are similar, regardless of the specific clinical problem that initiated the response.

While free amino acids released from the muscle get reincorporated back into muscle, muscle protein synthesis is further stimulated only marginally or not at all by traditional nutrition in the stress response. The stress response kills the appetite so much that it is hard to eat much food, and even when you do force down food or rely on traditional meal replacement beverages, you see little or no beneficial response. The problem is that there are so many EAAs available in the muscle as precursors for protein synthesis as a result of the accelerated protein breakdown that the rate of synthesis is already close to maximal. The absorption of EAAs after consumption of intact protein is slow and the extent of the increase in EAAs is not large, with the result that dietary protein is ineffective in stimulating synthesis because there is not enough of a change in the EAA concentrations in the muscle (**Figure 12.2**). The stress response causes severe *anabolic resistance*.

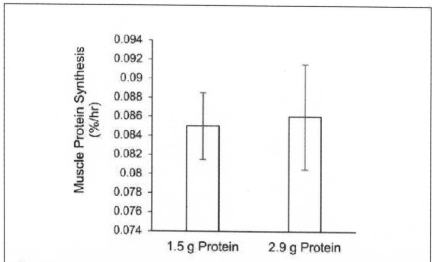

Figure 12.2. The stress response includes severe anabolic resistance of protein synthesis to the normal effects of dietary protein. An increase of dietary protein from 1.15 to 2.9 g protein/kg/day would normally increase muscle protein synthesis, but not in injured patients.

   In order for muscle protein synthesis to be further increased in the stress response, there must be an activation of the intracellular molecules involved in initiating protein synthesis. Remember mTOR, the "starter" that we discussed in relation to leucine and when we talked about anabolic resistance? Activation of mTOR can be accomplished by consumption of a supplement of free EAAs with a high proportion of leucine. The reason that free EAA mixtures containing a high proportion of leucine can activate the "starter" while EAAs from intact protein are ineffective is because the free EAAs are absorbed more rapidly, and the high-leucine formulation of free EAAs does not occur naturally in any intact protein. Consequently, the blood and then the muscle concentrations reach much higher peak concentrations and in the relative proportions required to maximally stimulate muscle protein synthesis. In addition, if enough EAAs are consumed, the concentrations will rise high enough to inhibit muscle protein breakdown. The combination of activating mTOR while inhibiting protein breakdown translates to an improvement in the net balance between protein synthesis and breakdown. To recap, consumption of a mixture of free EAAs with high leucine can slow the net loss of muscle protein whereas an intact protein in a meal or a meal replacement beverage is ineffective during physiological stress.

We discussed in some detail how the body uses different fuels to support different types of physical activity. In many ways, physiological stress is like exercise in that it affects the way the body uses different fuels. Carbohydrate and fat are the primary fuels that are involved. In this section, I'll briefly explain how stress affects substrate metabolism so that you can appreciate the metabolic basis for the recommendations of the EAASE program.

Insulin resistance is a hallmark of the stress response. This condition occurs when the hormone insulin loses its ability to stimulate glucose uptake from the blood by tissues such as muscle and liver. In a healthy person, insulin also prevents the liver from making and releasing glucose when it is not needed by muscle or other tissues. Insulin resistance prevents the liver from registering the message to stop producing glucose. As a result, blood glucose levels rise. The problem is made even worse by the fact that carbohydrate from foods that are eaten don't readily enter the muscle cells under these conditions. Instead of being used for energy production, much of the dietary glucose gets converted to fat, some of which is stored in the liver. Fat infiltration of the liver is a universal problem in critical illness and is another reason why so many metabolic problems accompany critical illness.

The way the body handles fat is also affected by physiological stress. Fat is stored in adipose tissue in the form of triglycerides, which are three fatty acids linked together. One of the main stress hormones is adrenaline and one of the actions of adrenaline is to mobilize fatty acids into the blood from stored triglycerides. The result is that there is an excessive amount of circulating fatty acids, more than is needed or can be used for energy. Extra dietary fat, then, is not efficiently used as an energy substrate, because there are already more than enough fatty acids in the blood to meet all requirements for energy. Consumption of dietary fat only adds to an already over-abundant supply of fatty acids in the blood, and these fatty acids also contribute to fat deposition in the liver.

As you can appreciate, it is a vexing situation that when the body has an increased demand for energy to deal with the challenges of physiological stress, the alterations in substrate metabolism due to the stress response make it difficult to obtain the normal benefit from dietary energy sources.

The Effects of Inactivity and the Stress Response

Illness, injury, and surgery bring about inactivity. If you are in the intensive care unit, you will likely be confined to bed. If you are over 65 years of age, you may be confined to bed in the hospital even when you are capable of walking because of concerns about stability and risk of a fall. After surgery, you are likely to be physically limited until incisions are healed and you have some degree of recovery. This is particularly true after orthopedic surgery. In all cases of serious illness, you probably don't feel much like exercising. As a result, the metabolic effects of the stress response are usually coupled with the catabolic effects of inactivity.

The interesting question, as a scientist, is "how do we know the degree to which inactivity amplifies the problems that occur due to physiological stress?" The answer was provided, in part, by a series of studies sponsored by the National Aeronautics and Space Agency (NASA). The lack of gravity during spaceflight

184

reduces the physical work of movement drastically, with the consequence that muscle loss during space flight can be severe. Enforced bed rest has been used by NASA as a model for the effects of the lack of gravity during space flight. We performed a number of these studies in which research volunteers were maintained at complete bed rest for a month or longer. Studies have not only been done in young, healthy subjects, but in older subjects as well. As you might expect, inactivity causes the opposite effects as exercise. Muscle mass and strength are reduced in bed rest. Bed rest also induces insulin resistance. The rate of deterioration of these factors is faster in older, as opposed to young subjects confined to bed rest.

By itself, inactivity is detrimental to muscle mass and function. When coupled with stress, bed rest amplifies the muscle loss. To try to better understand the role of inactivity, we did a study with healthy individuals who completed a bed rest trial. We then administered cortisol, a hormone that is considered one of the mediators of the stress response. We compared the response to cortisol infusion when subjects were ambulatory and had normal activity to their response to cortisol infusion during bed rest. Both bed rest and cortisol independently decrease muscle mass, strength and function but the loss of muscle is much more rapid when the two factors are combined. These studies taught us a great deal about metabolic changes brought about by serious illness or trauma. While the extent of physiological stress is less than in actual disease states such as cancer or severe injury, all of the same metabolic responses are evident.

Next, being practical scientists, we were interested in what treatments could help to minimize the loss of muscle and metabolic problems that occur in these conditions. One very interesting observation was that, allowing the subjects to perform a minimal amount of resistance exercise went a long way towards preserving muscle. We also tested the response to a balanced EAA mixture and found that the most effective therapy to slow the loss of muscle mass and strength in both young and older subjects when confined to bed rest is the consumption of multiple 15 g doses per day of EAA supplements. We also tested these treatments in a clinical trial in which EAAs were shown to speed recovery from hip or knee replacement. The important point relative to the EAASE Program is that the metabolic challenges presented by illness, injury and surgery are due to a combination of factors that result in the loss of muscle. Under these stressful conditions, multiple 15 g doses of EAA supplements were able to slow the loss of muscle mass, and strength (**Figure 12.3**).

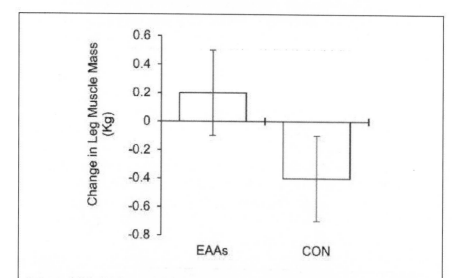

Figure 12.3. Prolonged (30 days) bed rest causes a significant loss of leg muscle mass and strength (controls, CON). Supplementation of the normal diet throughout the bed rest (EAAs) completely reversed the loss in muscle mass. EAA supplementation also improved several measures of physical function in older individuals confined to 10 days of bed rest.

Acute Response vs Recovery

The acute stress response can be considered the most severe phase. The word "acute" implies a short time, but the most serious phase of the stress response can last for months in some cases such as cancer. During the acute response, you can expect to lose body weight as well as muscle mass. You don't feel like eating, and conventional nutrition does not provide the desired beneficial effects. EAA supplements are uniquely suited for this phase of the response because they can be formulated to elicit a stimulation of muscle protein synthesis, even in the state of anabolic resistance as

186

well as the altered substrate metabolism of dietary carbohydrate and fat. The EAASE program does not provide specific recommendations for the acute.phase. While in general EAA supplements can provide nutritional benefit, there are so many different scenarios in the acute phase that it is not possible to provide a straight-forward program that will apply to everyone.

EAAs should play a central role in the recovery phase. Having lost significant muscle mass in the acute phase, you must pay attention to every aspect of your rehabilitation to avoid replacing the lost muscle with fat. The goal in the recovery phase is to maximally increase muscle mass while not significantly increasing fat mass. The recovery phase still presents challenges, as many of the metabolic responses in the acute phase are slow to recover in the recovery phase. Also, you won't feel like exercising, or you may actually be physically limited in performing exercise. Consequently, EAA supplements provide a unique stimulus to muscle protein synthesis. The specific details of the EAASE program for recovery are presented in the EAASE Program section.

Kidney Disease

The kidney is responsible for excreting waste products of metabolism. These include urea and ammonia, which are the end products of the metabolism of amino acids. Urea and ammonia are the principle forms in which the body gets rid of nitrogen from amino acid metabolism. Kidney disease is characterized by the failure to effectively clear these and other compounds from the blood. Kidney function is normally assessed by the ability to excrete creatinine (creatinine clearance). Creatinine is a by-product of the breakdown of muscle protein, and is normally completely filtered out of the blood passing through the kidney and excreted in the urine. Impaired kidney function is reflected by an elevation of the concentration of creatinine in the blood, reflecting decreased clearance. There are five stages of kidney disease that are determined clinically by the extent of impairment of creatinine clearance. Impaired excretion of urea and ammonia is also directly related to the stage of kidney disease. Elevations in the blood urea and ammonia concentrations in kidney disease exert a variety of adverse responses.

Many individuals have some degree of kidney disease. For example, approximately 60% of individuals over the age of 65 have some impairment in kidney function. While the symptoms of the early stages of impaired kidney function may not be severe, or even noticeable, the most severe stage of kidney disease (end stage) may be treated by either kidney transplant or the process of dialysis. Dialysis filters the blood to remove the excess urea and ammonia and other compounds normally excreted in the urine. It is extremely important to do whatever possible to avoid the need for dialysis. Dialysis runs the blood through a machine that filters the blood, thereby artificially doing the job of the kidney. For patients with end-stage kidney disease, dialysis is usually required multiple times per week and each session requires several hours. While dialysis can be life-saving for individuals without kidney function, there are adverse effects. Dialysis causes a robust inflammatory response that further antagonizes the physiological state of the patient. Also, dialysis is not as selective as a normally-functioning kidney in what is filtered. For example, amino acids in the blood are also filtered out by dialysis, which does not occur with normal kidney function. Kidney disease normally progresses slowly, even over a period of years. However, impaired kidney function can also occur in conjunction with other severe illnesses. Whether impaired kidney function is chronic or brought on suddenly by some other severe illness, it is important to prevent progression to end stage kidney failure.

Kidney disease induces the stress response characterized by loss of muscle mass and strength. The onset of the stress response in kidney disease is brought about in part by inflammation as well as hormonal responses including elevations in cortisol and epinephrine. In addition, the accumulation of urea and ammonia acidifies the blood, which has a direct inhibitory effect on muscle protein synthesis. The inhibition of protein synthesis by acidification of the blood because of impaired kidney function compounds the anabolic resistance that accompanies all serious illnesses. The result is a profound loss of muscle mass and strength in kidney disease that has many unfavorable consequences.

Anabolic resistance is difficult to overcome in any circumstance, but is particularly problematic in kidney disease. It would seem logical that the most effective dietary approach to anabolic resistance would be to consume a high protein diet. However, consumption of large amounts of dietary protein increases urea and ammonia production due to the metabolism of the absorbed amino acids that are not incorporated into protein. This is a high metabolic price to pay since anabolic resistance minimizes the effectiveness of protein intake. When kidney function is adequate, there is no problem excreting the extra urea and ammonia produced from the metabolism of the dietary protein. In fact, it is well established that high protein intake does not cause kidney failure when kidney function is normal. Unfortunately, a high protein diet amplifies the accumulation of urea and ammonia in the blood when kidney disease is established. Consequently, a low-protein diet is usually recommended to individuals with kidney disease. While a low protein diet minimizes the amount of urea and ammonia in the blood, a low protein diet in the setting of anabolic resistance accelerates the rate of muscle loss.

There is no circumstance in which the judicious use of dietary EAAs can provide more unique benefit than kidney disease. A brief review of the relationships between muscle protein metabolism, liver metabolism of amino acids released into the blood from muscle, and the excretion of urea and ammonia by the kidney, should make clear the role of dietary EAAs in lessening the devastating loss of muscle mass and function that normally occurs with kidney disease.

Muscle protein is in a constant state of turnover, meaning that protein is being broken down and releasing the component amino acids into the cell, while at the same time cellular amino acids are being incorporated into new protein (protein synthesis). An interchange of amino acids between the intracellular compartment and the blood also occurs continuously. The balance between protein synthesis and breakdown is determined by the rate of these various processes that are all occurring simultaneously.

The free amino acids in muscle cells are derived from the blood, protein breakdown, or, in the case of the non-essential amino acids (NEAAs) the production from other amino acids. In turn, the cellular amino acids may be incorporated into protein or released into the blood in their original form. Additionally, they may be partially metabolized, and the nitrogen transferred to form the NEAAs glutamine and alanine. Glutamine and alanine are the major vehicles that transport nitrogen from muscle to the liver, where the nitrogen is transferred to urea and ammonia and released into the blood. The blood is filtered by the kidney to selectively clear both urea and ammonia so they can be excreted in the urine.

Dietary EAAs stimulate the synthesis of new muscle protein. Since NEAAs comprise approximately half of muscle protein, and consumption of an EAA dietary supplement does not include NEAAs, the production of complete muscle protein requires that NEAAs be derived in part from protein breakdown. As a result, NEAA concentrations, including alanine and glutamine, are reduced by EAA consumption. Release of alanine and glutamine into the blood from muscle is correspondingly reduced. As a result of reduced flux of alanine and glutamine to the liver, the production of both urea and ammonia are reduced. Thus, EAA consumption stimulates muscle protein synthesis while lessening the burden on the kidney to excrete urea and ammonia. The devastating effect of the combination of anabolic resistance and reduced protein intake can be overcome with EAAs.

The relationships between muscle protein and amino acid metabolism, urea production in the liver, and urea excretion by the kidney are shown in **Figures 12.4 and 12.5**. Ammonia is not shown because it contributes much less than urea to the flux of nitrogen in the body.

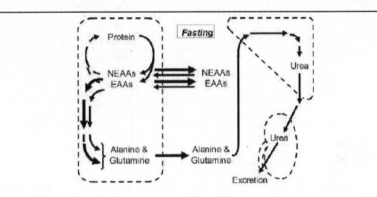

Figure 12.4. When amino acids are not being absorbed from the intestine (fasting state), the rate of muscle protein breakdown exceeds the rate of protein synthesis. The amino acids released from protein breakdown (both EAAs and NEAAs) are either released from muscle into the blood in their original form or partially metabolized to form alanine and glutamine. Alanine and glutamine travel to the liver via the blood, where they serve as primary precursors for the production of urea and ammonia in the liver. The resulting urea and ammonia are released into the blood, where they travel to the kidney for filtration of the blood and excretion in urine.

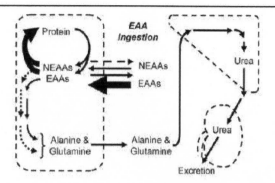

Figure 12.5. Consumption of dietary EAAs causes a net uptake of EAAs into muscle. Increased uptake of EAAs stimulates muscle protein synthesis. The NEAAs that are required for the production of complete protein are derived largely from a more efficient reutilization of the NEAAs released by protein breakdown. Increased reincorporation of NEAAs released by protein breakdown decreases the formation and release of alanine and glutamine, with a resulting decrease in urea production by the liver and decreased burden on the kidney to excrete urea and ammonia.

Metabolic Syndrome and Cardiovascular Health

Blood and Liver Fat

Metabolic syndrome is not a specific disease, but rather a group of risk factors for cardiovascular disease as well as diabetes. Metabolic syndrome is characterized by higher than normal levels of plasma triglycerides, blood pressure, and reduced insulin sensitivity. Other blood lipid values are also altered in metabolic syndrome. Triglycerides are three fatty acids hooked together by a glycerol molecule. An elevation in the blood concentration of triglycerides is closely tied to the level of very low density lipoproteins (VLDL) in the blood, since most triglycerides are carried in the blood VLDL. An elevation in triglycerides is also tied to an elevation in low density lipoproteins and a reduction in high density lipoproteins, the "good" fat in the blood. An elevation in blood triglycerides in particular may be used as a marker for an overall elevation in lipids that tend to cause arteriosclerosis.

There is a cycling of fatty acids from the adipose tissue to the liver and back to the adipose tissue that is primarily responsible for the triglycerides in the blood. The "free fatty acids" released into the blood from the triglyceride stored in adipose tissue are a major source of energy for most of the body. The free fatty acids are taken up in various tissues such as muscle and used for energy. However, fatty acids are released from adipose tissue at a rate that is greater than required for energy metabolism in other tissues. Under normal conditions, the liver clears the excess fatty acids from the blood and re-forms triglycerides. The liver triglycerides are then packaged with proteins to form VLDL particles, which are then secreted into the blood. The VLDL returns the triglyceride to the adipose tissue for storage. The triglycerides in the VLDL are broken down into fatty acids in the small blood vessels in the adipose tissue so that the fatty acids can be taken up. Once in the adipose tissue, triglycerides are reformed for storage. When the triglyceride in VLDL is broken down for uptake into adipose tissue, the particles become denser, and are termed low density lipoproteins (LDL). Thus, VLDL transports triglycerides in the blood from the liver to the adipose tissue, and LDL is the by-product of the uptake of the fatty acids from the triglycerides in the VLDL. The relationships between triglycerides, VLDL and LDL explain why an elevation in blood triglycerides can be used as a marker for an overall elevation in blood lipids.

Proteins (and thus amino acids) play a key role in two aspects of the cycling of fatty acids from adipose tissue to the liver and back to the adipose tissue. Triglycerides produced in the liver from the excess free fatty acids released from adipose tissue must combine with proteins to form lipoprotein particles for secretion into the blood. The protein ApoB plays a key regulatory role in this regard, but other proteins are involved as well. If there is a deficiency in ApoB synthesis in the liver, the production and secretion of VLDL will be limited. Limited ApoB synthesis will therefore lead to accumulation of triglycerides in the liver. Triglyceride accumulation in the liver contributes to disruption of metabolic processes in the liver, particularly the normal action of insulin. Elevated liver triglyceride content can also be a precursor of fibrosis and ultimately cirrhosis.

The second way in which proteins affect the cycling of fatty acids and triglycerides is in the small blood vessels perfusing adipose tissue. A protein called *lipoprotein lipase* is responsible for breaking apart the triglyceride in the VLDL so the resulting free fatty acids can be taken up by adipose tissue. The intact triglyceride cannot be directly taken up by adipose tissue, so an inadequate supply of lipoprotein lipase will lead to an increase in blood VLDL concentrations.

Conventional pharmacological therapy to reduce triglycerides includes statins, nicotinic acid (niacin) and fenofibrate. Statins are mostly designed to lower LDL levels by increasing their uptake and metabolism by the liver. Statins may also lower triglycerides by limiting VLDL production, but generally only cause a decrease of 10-20 %. Niacin directly inhibits the release of free fatty acids from the adipose tissue, thereby decreasing liver uptake of fatty acids, and as a result reducing the rate of triglyceride formation in the liver. Fenofibrate activates the clearance of triglycerides from circulating VLDL by improving the ability of mitochondria to oxidize fatty acids.

All pharmacological treatments of lipid disorders have potential adverse side effects. Statins can deplete CoQ10 (an important cofactor of certain physiological reactions), which results in muscle soreness. Both niacin and fenofibrate can impair normal liver function and may cause itching and rashes, particularly in older individuals.

EAAs and Plasma and Liver Lipids

Supplementation of the diet with EAA-based formulations, either in combination with protein or as pure EAAs, has consistently been shown to lower blood triglycerides, total cholesterol, VLDL and LDL. In addition, liver triglyceride was lowered approximately 50% by 4 weeks of EAA therapy in older individuals. The reduction in liver fat was associated with an improvement in insulin sensitivity. There may be several mechanisms involved, but most prominently, dietary EAA supplementation stimulates the synthesis of ApoB, and therefore enables more efficient transport of triglycerides from the liver back to the adipose tissue for storage. This effect reduces accumulation of triglycerides in the liver. EAA supplementation also increases lipoprotein lipase activity at the adipose tissue, so that uptake of fatty acids into adipose tissue is improved. Both components of the cycling of fatty acids from adipose tissue to the liver and back to the adipose tissue are thus enhanced by EAAs, with the consequence of reduction in both liver and circulating lipids.

There are two important aspects of EAA supplementation. First, in contrast to pharmacological approaches, there are no known adverse responses to dietary EAA supplementation. Dietary EAAs are not only naturally-occurring nutrients, but they are the only macronutrients that are mandatory for survival. Dietary EAAs can beneficially impact blood and liver lipids without the potential adverse effects of pharmacological therapy.

Secondly, the mechanisms of action of dietary EAAs complement the mechanisms of actions of drugs commonly used for lowering lipids. The wide use of statins reflects their effectiveness in lowering LDL, but statins have minimal effects of triglycerides. The addition of dietary EAA supplementation to statin therapy will cause further reductions in all lipids, particularly triglycerides, than can be achieved with statins alone. Niacin can effectively limit the release of fatty acids from adipose tissue. The combination of niacin and dietary EAAs will not only reduce the release of fatty acids from adipose tissue (niacin effect), but also increase the efficiency of the transport of liver triglycerides as VLDL back to the adipose tissue for reincorporation into stored triglyceride (EAA effect). The combination of dietary EAAs and fenofibrate will improve the oxidation of fatty acids (fenofibrate) and also reduce liver and blood triglycerides by stimulation of ApoB synthesis and activation of lipoprotein lipase (EAA effect).

Dietary EAAs play an important role in optimizing liver and blood lipid levels whether alone or in combination with traditional drug therapy.

Blood Pressure

Elevated blood pressure is a risk factor for a cardiovascular event. The nature of high blood pressure is easy to envision if you think of fluid being pumped through a tube of a certain diameter, and then the diameter of the tube is reduced. In order to get the same amount of fluid through a narrowed tube, the pressure generated by the pump must increase. This is in essence what happens in the case of high blood pressure. The heart must pump out blood into a vascular system that is functionally narrowed. Narrowing of the vascular system can occur from atherosclerosis, and/or the lack of the ability of the vessels to relax (dilate). Nitric oxide (NO) is a key regulator of blood pressure and the amount of blood that perfuses different tissues and organs. NO is a potent dilator of the vascular system.

NO is produced in the body from arginine. Arginine is not a true essential amino acid, as it can be produced in the body. However, arginine is considered "conditionally" essential because it often is not produced at a sufficient rate for optimal metabolic function. This situation occurs in a number of diseases and in natural circumstances, such as aging. Insufficient arginine results in inadequate NO, and is often related to hypertension (high blood pressure). Supplemental dietary arginine increases NO production, and as a result can decrease blood pressure.

There are some limitations to providing supplemental dietary arginine. In large doses, arginine can upset the stomach. Also, the liver clears arginine from the blood very effectively. Since dietary arginine that is absorbed from the intestine passes through the liver before it reaches the rest of the body, a large amount of arginine may be needed to raise the peripheral blood concentration sufficiently to stimulate the production of enough NO to markedly reduce the blood pressure. Citrulline may be used as a dietary supplement to increase the arginine concentration in peripheral blood. Citrulline is an amino acid that is not part of the body's protein. Rather, it is a by-product of the production of NO from arginine. In a cyclical reaction, citrulline then serves as a precursor for the production of more arginine. Since the production of arginine from citrulline occurs in the kidney, the plasma concentration of arginine increases quite rapidly when citrulline is given as a dietary supplement. Interestingly, arginine concentration in peripheral blood increases to a greater extent when citrulline is given than when an equal amount of arginine is consumed. Whether arginine or citrulline is consumed, NO production is stimulated and elevated blood pressure may be reduced.

Heart Failure

Heart failure develops when the heart becomes weakened and consequently is compromised in its ability to contract, relax, or both. Impaired heart function leads to reduced exercise capacity, which in turn leads to progressive muscle weakness and a vicious cycle of sedentary behavior, weight gain, and subsequent

197

development of metabolic abnormalities and sarcopenia. There are many stages of heart failure, and most individuals over the age of 65 suffer from at least the mildest form of heart failure. Heart failure is a serious condition that can greatly limit physical function, decrease quality of life, and can be a cause of death.

There are two principal forms of heart failure, both of which involve reduced pumping capacity of the heart. Most commonly, heart failure involves reduced force of ejection. Heart failure may also result from an impaired ability of the heart to relax, which is important for the heart to fill adequately before it contracts again. This latter form of heart failure is the predominant form of heart failure. There is a wide range of potential causes of heart failure, including the natural process of aging.

Regardless of the specific underlying cause or type of heart failure, there are common pathophysiological responses. Most prominently, heart failure limits exercise capacity and causes shortness of breath, fatigue and reduces muscle strength. Taken together, these symptoms impair physical function, which leads to sedentary behavior and insulin resistance. Another complication of long-standing heart failure is loss of muscle mass due to anabolic resistance.

Pharmacological treatment of heart failure predominantly targets the improvement of the performance of the heart. Heart failure may be treated with varying degrees of success with a variety of drugs. However, treating heart failure pharmacologically may be quite complex in the elderly. More than 50% of individuals over age 65 with heart failure have at least four other significant medical issues, and these may complicate therapy of heart failure. Adverse responses to pharmacological therapy are common, including further impairment of muscle function.

The limitations that arise in physical function in heart failure originate with decreased capacity of the heart. While the heart is a muscle and we could expect that EAA supplementation would improve the strength of the heart muscle, there are no studies that document this effect. Loss of muscle mass and function also

198

contribute to the debilitation of heart failure, and we know that dietary EAA supplementation can have a beneficial effect on those factors. As in all cases of anabolic resistance, formulations of EAAs can stimulate the synthesis of new protein more effectively than intact protein. When compared to a popular meal replacement specifically promoted for heart function, consumption of an EAA formulation designed to overcome anabolic resistance induced a much greater net gain in the production of protein **(Figure 12.6)**. Increased net protein synthesis is the metabolic basis for increased muscle mass and strength. Stimulation of net protein synthesis by dietary EAAs has led to improved physical function over time in a variety of circumstances.

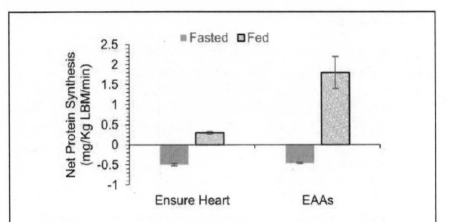

Figure 12.6. EAAs overcome anabolic resistance in heart failure. Elderly individuals with heart failure were studied on two occasions. Following an overnight fast, they consumed either one serving of Ensure Heart (9 g protein, 220 kcal) or one 11 g serving (44 kcal) of an EAA formulation. Ensure Heart had little effect on protein synthesis, breakdown, or the balance between protein synthesis and breakdown (net protein synthesis). The minimal response to Ensure Heart reflects anabolic resistance. In contrast, EAAs stimulated protein synthesis, inhibited breakdown, and improved net protein synthesis to a far greater extent than Ensure Heart. The total increase in net protein synthesis after EAAs was 21.7 g, as compared to the intake of 11 g of EAAs. The net production of more protein than EAAs were consumed was possible because the NEAAs comprise about 60% of the protein in the body, and when EAAs are provided, the NEAAs in the newly synthesized protein are recycled from protein breakdown.

Essentials

- The metabolic response to serious illness and disease, trauma and surgery are similar and can be called the *stress response.*
- Muscle loss occurs at a rapid rate in the stress response, and the muscle protein is resistant to the normal anabolic effect of dietary protein. This is called *anabolic resistance.*
- Substrate metabolism is altered in the stress response. Coupled with anabolic resistance to dietary protein, conventional nutrition is of limited benefit.
- Inactivity amplifies the loss of muscle mass in the stress response.
- Loss of body weight and muscle mass in the acute stress response is inevitable. The challenge in the recovery stage is to regain lost muscle mass without a significant gain in fat mass. EAAs play a key role in accomplishing this goal.
- EAA formulations can overcome anabolic resistance and decrease the loss of muscle protein due to the stress response.
- Dietary EAAs are ideally suited for nutritional support of kidney disease. EAAs stimulate muscle protein synthesis while decreasing the metabolic demands on the kidney by causing recycling of NEAAs into protein. The efficient reutilization of NEAAs limits their breakdown and the resulting production of urea and ammonia.
- Dietary EAAs can improve symptoms of the metabolic syndrome that are risk factors for the development of cardiovascular disease and diabetes.
- The anabolic resistance in heart failure can be overcome by dietary EAA formulations.

SECTION 3. THE EAASE PROGRAM

Fundamentals of the EAASE Plan

The EAASE program is designed to work for everyone. In this section, I will lay out for you basic information about the basic program. The specific examples I provide in this section are relevant to all circumstances but specifically directed towards young to middle-aged healthy individuals who want to benefit from the combination of the optimal diet, EAA supplements, and exercise. In subsequent sections, I will deal with how the basic program should be modified for special circumstances. In all circumstances, I will discuss how I have relied on solid principles of protein and amino acid science that have been highlighted in the previous chapters.

The EAASE program takes the approach that the body in balance must achieve optimal functioning of muscle, heart, organs, and brain. The core strategies of diet, EAA supplements and exercise will build muscle and improve heart health as well as provide essential substrates to optimize brain and liver function. While each individual component of the program will provide benefits, I highly recommend that you strive to incorporate all three elements. Like a three-legged stool, the EAA supplements in combination with a diet emphasizing high-quality protein and physical activity work synergistically to amplify the individual effects of the three elements. This section focuses on the three core

201

aspects of the EAASE program: diet, exercise, and EAA supplements. Applications of the EAASE program for specific conditions will follow.

The Basic Diet

Dietary Protein Intake

Throughout the book, I have emphasized the central role of muscle in health and disease and the way in which consumption of adequate EAAs promotes muscle mass, strength and function. The most important aspect of diet in the EAASE plan is the amount and profile of the EAAs contained in the dietary protein. However, it is unrealistic to try to keep track of all the different EAAs in your dietary protein. To simplify, the plan is based on the percentage of calories consumed as high quality protein. I think you will find that the actual implementation of this strategy is pretty straightforward and offers a lot of flexibility in food choices. In the interest of providing you the basis for determining how much protein and the types of protein to eat, I present some mathematical calculations and examples. These calculations are mainly described for you to see where my dietary recommendations come from. The EAASE program is designed so you don't need to perform all of these calculations to plan your diet. There are multiple options to figuring out your personal dietary goals and these will be discussed. The overriding purpose of this section is to make it clear why high-quality proteins and EAAs provide the foundation for the diet and the program, and to help you achieve the optimal intake in the form of dietary protein.

High quality proteins are defined by the amount of EAAs per gram of protein, as well as how the profile of EAAs corresponds to the dietary requirements (RDAs) for each amino acid. Account is also taken of digestibility in the quantification of protein quality. Protein quality is quantified by the Digestible Indispensable Amino Acid Score (DIAAS), and a score over 100 is considered to be a high quality protein.

The EAASE program is based on the amount of EAAs you consume every day. The specific amount of EAAs you derive from dietary protein can differ according to your individual needs. The general target for the diet is to include at least 25% of the calories as high quality proteins. This amount of protein intake is well within established dietary recommendations, and no health concerns have been documented when as much as 35% or more of the calories are consumed as protein. Food sources of high-quality protein (as determined by DIAAS) are generally animal-based, including dairy products, eggs, meat, fish, and poultry. The diet of most Americans is "omnivorous" meaning a mixture of animal and plant foods are consumed. If you prefer to rely extensively or entirely on plant-based protein, I will show you how to achieve your optimal protein nutrition.

Determining Your Dietary Intake of Protein and Calories

The EAASE diet goal is to eat 25% of your calories as high-quality proteins. It is therefore necessary to have a pretty good idea of how many calories you eat in a day so that you can figure out 25% of that amount. If you have ever dieted to lose weight, you may have an idea of how many calories you consume on average and maybe even what percentage of those calories come from protein. If you did this, you know that counting calories is tedious and often not straight-forward. Consequently, counting calories is not a requirement of EAASE. If you follow the entire program, you will find it easy to naturally maintain energy balance without counting calories. We do, however, have to find some way to plan a diet that delivers the optimal amount of protein in terms of the percentage of total caloric intake. There are plenty of diets and menu plans that you can follow through books and websites to meet the target of protein comprising 25% of caloric intake. This may sound like a simple solution but it often takes a lot of effort, sacrifice, and money to buy the foods, prepare the recipes, and stick to assigned menus of most diet plans. The EAASE basic diet plan is based on figuring out the best approach for you personally, rather than dictating specific food choices.

The first step I recommend is to take a look at your current diet before revising it. Realize that making a huge change in what you are currently doing is probably not realistic. You may recognize that you need to improve your diet, but that should be accomplished using a dietary pattern that you will adhere to for years, not just the next month or so while the change is exciting and new. Consequently, you need to base your dietary pattern, to the extent possible, on foods that you like to eat. This is why I recommend not following someone else's dietary plan, but figuring out one that accomplishes the EAASE goal with regard to protein intake that works for you.

There are a number of options available to quantify your current dietary intake. The best one for you depends upon the level of detail you desire. If you want a good, quantitative estimate of your calorie intake and macronutrient breakdown, you will have to keep some form of a diet record. From a diet record, you can calculate how much of each general category of nutrients you are eating on average. There are a variety of computer programs and apps designed to help you record and analyze your food intake. Another option is to enlist the help of a dietician or nutritionist to calculate your nutrient intake from your diet record.

Diet records track your food intake for different lengths of time; there are forms on the internet for 24-hour, 3-day, and 7-day food diaries. Each has its strengths and weaknesses. For a 24-hour recall, you will describe everything you consumed over the past 24 hours. The advantage to this approach is there is no conscious awareness of recording what is eaten when food selections are made. Therefore, the foods and the amounts eaten are likely to be representative of usual intake. Disadvantages of the diet recall approach include under-reporting because you simply forget food or drinks that were eaten, or you don't recall the exact amounts consumed. Also, the particular day chosen may not be representative of the usual intake. Everyone has days when circumstances and events interfere with normal food choices. The 3-Day record requires that you record everything that is eaten for 3 days, usually including a week-end day and 2 week days to try to account for different patterns of eating on work days versus vacation days. A 7-day record documents the entire food intake for 7 consecutive days. The disadvantage to these approaches is the likelihood that the act of recording all that is eaten will influence the decision whether or not to eat the food. You may want to eat a second helping but decide not to because you know that the total amount of food you've eaten will need to be recorded. Dietary records are very time consuming, not just time spent recording the amount and type of food/meal eaten, but even more so in analyzing the nutrient contribution of all foods eaten.

The primary database to convert various foods into calories and individual nutrients is the United States Department of Agriculture (USDA) Food Composition database (https://ndb.nal.usda.gov/ndb/search). There are many websites and apps now that link to this database to make the process of diet analysis easier. While many mixed foods are listed (for example, pepperoni pizza), sometimes a more complicated or unique recipe needs to be broken down and each component analyzed.

The decision to do a full analysis of your current diet is up to you. Keep in mind that the EAASE diet is focused on the percentage of energy eaten as protein, so exact amounts of carbohydrate and fat do not need to be tracked unless that information is of interest to you. The popularity of the various diet-analysis websites is testimony to the fact that many people like to break down their diets to analyze them in detail. In my experience, the exercise is often unproductive because of imprecision in record keeping, uncertainty in determining the exact amount of different foods consumed, and (most importantly) the failure to distinguish protein sources by quality. The computer programs do not distinguish the quality of protein, and the EAASE program is based on the consumption of high quality protein.

Determining How Much Protein to Consume Without all the Record Keeping

A reasonable estimate of a diet plan that provides approximately 25% of calories as protein can be made fairly easily without all the record keeping or diet planning. The first step is to determine how many total calories you should consume each day. Then it's just a matter of multiplying the total calorie intake by 0.25 to get the calories from protein.

Unless you are gaining or losing weight at a significant rate, your total energy intake is defined by your energy expenditure plus or minus a small number of calories. There are several easy calculations to determine your total energy expenditure (and thus your dietary caloric requirement). First, calculate your basal metabolic rate. **Table 1** shows the Harris-Benedict equations for estimating the basal metabolic rate in men and women. Your basal energy expenditure is how much energy you need to stay alive as you lie in bed after not eating all night.

Table 1. Estimating Energy Expenditure

Step 1. Calculate basal metabolic rate:
Men: BMR = 66 + {6.23 x wt (lbs) + (12.7 x ht (in)} – (6.8 x age (yrs))

Women: BMR = 655 + {4.35 x wt (lbs) + (4.7 x ht (in)} – (4.7 x age (yrs))

Step 2. Estimate activity factor:

Low activity	1.4-1.6
Active	1.6-1.9
Very active	2.0-2.5

Once you calculate your basal metabolic rate, total energy expenditure is obtained by multiplying the basal metabolic rate by the appropriate activity factor. The activity factor will generally range from 1.2 (sedentary) to 2 (organized daily exercise, or a very active lifestyle). If you are participating in an endurance sport, or have a physically demanding job, the factor is likely to be even higher. You actually don't even need a calculator since there are multiple websites that only require you to type in your weight, height, age, and activity level (http://manytools.org/handy/bmr-calculator is one example).

Once you estimate your total energy expenditure you know your energy requirement, since energy intake = energy expenditure unless you are gaining or losing weight.

The next step is to calculate the protein calories you need to consume each day. This equation is simple. Multiply the total energy expenditure value that you calculated for yourself by 0.25 (the fraction of the diet as high quality protein). This number represents the target goal of protein calories. Determining the food sources that will add up to the desired amount of calories as protein will require some work initially. Nutrition labels provide the amount of protein in grams per listed serving. You can calculate the protein calories by multiplying the number of protein grams by 4 (~4kcal/gram protein). Information for foods without nutrition labels can be found in the USDA Nutrient Data Base which lists many thousands of foods.

To get started, **Table 2** presents some representative examples of common protein food sources. The column labeled "Energy as protein" in Table 2 tells you how many calories as protein you are getting from the food source you eat. The values in this table are all for one ounce of the food so that you can easily see the differences between the various protein sources. We will calculate the protein calories for a 36 year old woman who is 5'6" tall (66"), weighing 140 lbs, and is moderately active (performs some kind of activity every day, but otherwise works at a desk). The goal is to consume about 25% of calories as high quality protein.

Table 2. Caloric Equivalents Calculated from Data in USDA Nutrient Data Base: (https//ndb.nal.usda.gov)

Protein Food Source	Energy as Protein (kcal/oz)	Total Energy (kcal/oz)	% Energy as Protein
A. Animal-Based Food Source			
Beef (90% lean ground)	28	51	57
Egg (whole, poached)	14	40	35
Milk (1% milk fat)	5	13	38
Yogurt (low fat)	18	29	62
Lamb (composite)	28	40	70
Venison	34	42	81
Pork (ham)	33	59	56
Pork (tenderloin)	23	32	72
B. Plant-Based Food Sources			
Soy Beans	13	41	32
Kidney Beans	6	23	25
Chickpeas	8	39	20
Mixed Nuts	23	170	13
Seeds (sunflower)	23	165	14

First, calculate basal energy expenditure:

Basal energy expenditure (female) = 655 + {(4.35 x wt (lbs) + (4.7 x ht (in)} − (4.7 x age (yrs)) = 655 + 609 + 310 − 169 = 1,405 kcal per day.

Next, multiply basal energy expenditure by the appropriate activity factor to calculate total energy expenditure.

In this example, we will estimate the activity factor to be 1.7:

Total energy expenditure = 1,405 kcal/day x 1.7 = 2,388 kcal per day.

These values are estimates, so we will round it off to 2,400 kcal per day.

To determine the target for dietary protein calories (i.e., 25% of total caloric intake), multiply 2,400 kcal/day by 0.25 = 600 kcal/day of dietary protein.

Once you have the calories per day of high quality protein in your diet, you can make a dietary plan based on the caloric equivalents of the protein food sources in your diet. The values shown in Table 2, along with additional data, can be found in the USDA nutrient data base for just about any possible food source. Table 2 shows values per ounce but the database offers various options for serving size consistent with how the food is usually consumed (for example, one cup of milk). Obviously, a dietary plan that uses only the items listed in Table 2 will be limited, so please realize it is just for example to show you how to formulate your own diet.

An example of a dietary plan adding up to 600 kcal of protein taken from Table 2 is shown in **Table 3**. 600 protein calories is the target. However, we don't generally eat pure protein. To plan an actual diet, we have to consider the actual food sources that contain the protein. For example, we don't eat egg protein in pure form, but we eat eggs that contain egg protein, along with other nutrients as well.

Table 3. Example of dietary meal plan.

Breakfast:	Protein kcal	Total kcal
2 eggs	46	131
Yogurt	72	116
Total Breakfast:	118 kcal	247 kcal
Lunch:		
Ham (6 oz)	198	353
1 cup milk	40	105
Total Lunch:	238 kcal	458 kcal
Dinner:		
Beef patty (8 oz)	224	431
½ cup milk	20	54
Total Dinner:	244 kcal	485 kcal

Breakfast + Lunch + Dinner = 600 total protein kcal; 1,190 total kcal

Table 2 is provided just to give you an idea of different protein density of food and how the values are derived. If you use the nutrient database or a program or app linked to it, you will see that caloric values will vary depending on how a food is prepared, the particular brand, or the serving size. In our sample menu, the database will give us the total calories for one large egg and the grams of protein in one egg. Two eggs provide a total of 131 kcal and ~12 grams of protein to obtain 46 kcal of protein. Using this approach for each protein food source represented in Table 3, we can calculate the total calories as protein food sources. The total calories provided by these foods to obtain the target protein calories is 1,190 kcals. The remaining calories to meet the daily energy intake is 1,210 kcal (2,400 − 1,190 = 1,210). The somewhat Spartan menu plan presented can be enhanced by healthy carbohydrate/fat food sources; juice and fruit, bread and vegetables, maybe even dessert, to meet the energy total for the day.

There are a number of interesting things that you can take from this example. First, you don't have to plan every aspect of your diet to meet the protein calorie goal. Over time, you will get familiar with food choices that get you to your target. Also, the numbers here are not an exact science. Some days, your diet may only reach 22% protein whereas on others, it may add up to 30% or more. This variation is fine as long as, on average, you hit the 25% target. More importantly, this example demonstrates the importance of high-quality proteins to meet the goal in a calorically efficient manner. Even with the high protein density in the foods selected in the example in Table 3, almost half of caloric intake is in the form of protein food sources.

Plant-based proteins can contribute to your total protein and EAA intake, but they are not as efficient on a calorie per ounce basis. If you substitute plant-based for animal-based protein food sources, you will need to eat roughly twice the calories in the form of the plant-based protein food to get the same EAA intake as from animal-based protein foods. This difference is due to protein density as well as the DIAASs of plant-based proteins, which are less than half the animal based protein food sources, based not only on EAA composition but also digestibility.

It is helpful to see how these things play out by considering examples. For most people, protein food sources are a combination of animal- and plant-based protein food sources. Let's drop the yogurt for breakfast and make up the protein energy with mixed nuts in granola, and drop the ham for lunch, and substitute a vegetable broth soup with kidney beans. For the amount of protein to remain the same with these two substitutions, we would need 3 oz of mixed nuts (69 protein kcal) to substitute for the yogurt, which is not too unreasonable. However, we would need 33 oz, or 2 pounds, of kidney beans to provide the equivalent protein as the ham. If you further consider that the DIAAS of kidney bean protein is half the value of pork protein (reflecting the EAA content, profile and digestibility), then you would need twice that amount of kidney beans to replace the amount of EAAs that you have dropped from your meal plan by substituting the kidney beans for ham. That would be 4 pounds of kidney beans to substitute for a thick slice of ham. Not only would that be a lot of kidney beans to eat, but you would be getting a lot of non-protein calories as well. When you add the extra calories resulting from the kidney beans and nuts to the amount of calories from the other protein food sources, the total calories of all protein food sources would be more than 80% of total calories. This would leave you little flexibility with the remainder of your diet.

Granted, many foods provide some amount of protein. For example, the oats in the granola provide 5 grams of protein per one cup serving. One could argue that throughout the day, these small amounts from "non-protein" food sources add up. However, these sources of protein do not contribute to your "high-quality" protein intake. The point of high-quality protein is to optimize EAA intake. The original food group designation emphasized meats, fish, poultry, eggs and dairy products as the "protein foods". If you look at the column labeled "percent energy as protein" in Table 2, you can see that eating a mixture of plant-based protein food sources would provide less than 25% of total caloric intake as protein, even if you ate only these protein food sources. When you consider the low DIAAS values of these proteins, you will be far short of the optimal EAA nutrition eating only plant-based proteins.

From these simple calculations, it should be clear in quantitative terms why the regular diet component of the EAASE plan specifies "high-quality" dietary proteins. Lower quality proteins are not only deficient in EAAs, but they also are contained in food sources that tend to not be completely digested and contain a relatively low percentage of protein relative to total calories. Vegan diets must rely heavily on soy products given the relatively high DIAAS of soy protein amongst plant proteins. Lacto-ovo vegetarian diets (allowing dairy and egg proteins) provide much more flexibility in terms of non-protein calories than a vegan diet, but still present problems in achieving optimal EAA intake.

214

The goal of this section is not to recommend against diets with restrictions against animal-based proteins, but to demonstrate quantitatively the challenge you will face with this approach in terms of consuming the optimal amount of dietary EAAs through your basic diet.

Putting Your Diet Plan into Action

The previous section should give you some insight into the fact that to meet a dietary goal of 25%, some attention to planning a dietary pattern to follow is important, at least as you get started. Some people like to follow a prescribed diet and menu plan. The popularity of high protein diets has led to many commercially available plans and books that offer recipes and complete menus designed to provide up to 30% of calories as protein. These resources may be utilized to help in achieving the protein goal for the EAASE program, but keep in mind that you do not want to follow recommendations for losing weight unless that is a goal. Also, the internet provides many useful websites offering tools, databases and on-line worksheets to help in diet planning. This information can be helpful in planning menus or just getting a feel for foods that target the optimal amount of dietary protein consumption.

It is important to remember that the focus of the EAASE program regarding protein in the diet relates to the EAAs that are provided in high quality proteins. Therefore, if you have diet preferences or restrictions that limit the amount of animal-based protein foods you eat, it is doubly important to match complementary proteins in your meals and make every effort to focus on eating enough protein to account for the limited bioavailability of plant proteins. Even with complementary proteins, it is likely that you will fall short of the target for EAA consumption without animal-based protein foods in your dietary pattern. Overcoming shortages in high-quality dietary EAAs is one of the ways in which EAA supplements can play an important role in achieving optimal EAA nutrition.

The Non-Protein Components of Your Diet

The principal aspect of the regular diet plan of the EAASE program is the amount of calories you consume in the form of high quality protein. This leaves flexibility for the rest of the diet, assuming you haven't "used up" all your calories with protein food sources. The ideal ratio of macronutrients is an individual thing, depending upon a person's genetic makeup, activity level, and food preferences. The EAASE program is intended to be a plan for life, so it is up to you to decide how to fill in the remaining 30-60% of calories not included in your protein food sources. We are basically talking about macronutrient choices and the options are simple: carbohydrate, fat, and possibly, alcohol.

Many books have been written about both the benefits and evils of dietary carbohydrates and fats (as well as alcohol). It is beyond the scope of the EAASE plan to go into your non-protein food choices in great detail, except when relevant to a specific circumstance (discussed in the following section).

Carbohydrate foods are implicated in some adverse health outcomes including elevated triglycerides and insulin insensitivity. High fat foods are calorie dense and, for some individuals, may worsen blood lipid profiles. If your current diet favors carbohydrates over fats, and you have no specific complications that you can attribute directly to your food choices, then it is fine to continue eating the same amount of carbohydrates. Physically active people especially will function better with adequate carbohydrate intake to optimize muscle glycogen for support of aerobic exercise and participation in sporting activities. Your carbohydrate intake should come largely from whole grains, fruits and vegetables. To the extent possible, your fat intake should focus on the newly recognized "healthy fats" including omega three fatty acids, mono-unsaturated fats and some poly-unsaturated fats. If you are consuming a significant amount of animal-based protein food sources, you will inevitably be consuming saturated fats along with the protein. Research is still evolving on the benefits/adverse effects of consuming saturated fats.

Cutting back on carbohydrate foods like bread, pastas, and sugary baked goods in your diet will help in weight management and overall health. These types of products provide little nutritional benefit beyond the calories they provide. Particularly beneficial results will be obtained if protein foods replace these types of carbohydrates. While a modest amount of alcohol consumption is not a problem, alcohol should not constitute a large portion of your caloric intake.

EAA Supplements

Why EAA Supplements?

EAA supplements play a central role in the EAASE program because of the importance of obtaining a specific profile and amount of EAAs to optimize muscle, heart, liver, and brain function. Throughout the book, I have stressed that formulations containing all the EAAs can target specific responses while maintaining the necessary balance of all the EAAs in the blood needed to maintain all the duties of the EAAs. Furthermore, the free EAAs in a supplement are absorbed more quickly and completely than possible with any intact protein, thereby providing a unique anabolic signal to the muscle and other organs and tissues.

EAA dietary supplements provide two main physiological benefits. When taken between meals the supplemental EAAs maintain a high rate of muscle protein turnover and stop the loss of muscle protein that occurs in the absence of food intake. A relatively small dose of EAAs (3-7 grams) can accomplish this goal. The second benefit of EAA supplements is that they can make up for inadequacies in the EAA composition of your regular diet.

The EAASE program recommends that, in most circumstances, 25% or more of the calories you eat are high quality proteins. The previous section gave detailed examples of what is involved in achieving this goal. Not everyone will succeed in consuming the recommended amount of high quality protein. This is particularly true if you prefer to eat only a small amount of animal-based protein food, or if you adhere to a vegetarian or vegan diet. If you are in this group, it is especially important that you use EAA supplements. Most EAA supplements are derived from vegan sources, so they can be used without disrupting your dietary commitment. With a vegetarian or vegan diet you are eating less than the ideal amount of EAAs in the form of high quality animal protein, but it is possible to make up for this shortfall by consuming more EAAs in the form of supplements. The amount of EAAs you need to consume as supplements depends on the extent to which you are missing your goal intake of high quality protein.

Provision of only the EAAs offers a metabolic advantage since the reutilization of NEAAs is amplified, thereby minimizing the oxidation of excess amino acids and consequent production of urea and ammonia. The other key aspect of an EAA supplement is that it adds to the overall nutrient intake but does not displace regular nutrition or meals. Finally, an EAA supplement optimizes the EAA profile of the blood with a negligible intake of calories and without effect on the response to normal dietary intake.

Muscle is a Primary Target of EAA Supplements

The most appropriate formulation of EAAs will depend on your particular circumstance. Specific cases (i.e., weight loss, catabolic states, athletic training, etc.) are dealt with in detail in the individual chapters. Regardless of the circumstance, muscle is always a target of EAA supplements. Recall that when regular meals are not being absorbed (post-absorptive state), the muscle protein is breaking down to supply EAAs for other tissues to maintain their rates of synthesis. An EAA supplement can be taken between meals to reverse the breakdown of muscle protein that would otherwise be occurring. The EAAs in a dietary supplement not only prevent the net loss of muscle protein, but they also maintain a higher rate of muscle protein turnover, which is the metabolic basis of improved physical function. It is important that all EAAs are present to provide the necessary precursors to produce new muscle protein.

While benefits of EAA supplements for the liver, heart and brain are generally of less concern for healthy, young and middle-aged individuals than promotion of muscle synthesis, the same balanced mixture of EAAs that promotes muscle protein synthesis will also promote heart and liver health and help to maintain the desired level of brain neurotransmitters.

Profile of EAAs

At this point, you probably wonder exactly what I mean by EAA supplements. One of the great things about EAA supplements is that they can be formulated to exact specifications for different circumstances. In that sense, you should appreciate that when I have referred to EAAs in the general sense I am assuming that the formulation of EAAs is targeting the specific circumstance of interest.

While there are almost limitless different possible profiles of EAAs, there are a few general principles that dictate the basic nature of the profile. Since the primary target is muscle, then a starting point will always be the profile of EAAs needed to provide precursors in the exact profile contained in muscle protein. The profile of EAAs in human skeletal muscle is shown in **Table 4**.

Table 4. EAA profile in human skeletal muscle.	
Amino Acid	**% of Total EAAs**
Histidine	6.2
Isoleucine	10.7
Leucine	21.2
Lysine	20.4
Methionine	4.5
Phenylalanine	8.2
Threonine	13.6
Valine	15.3

While duplicating the profile of skeletal muscle would seem like a logical place to start for the formulation of EAAs to stimulate muscle protein synthesis, it turns out some tweaking is necessary. If you give EAAs in the profile shown in Table 4, the increase in availability of EAAs inside the muscle cells will not reflect the proportions you gave. For one thing, the muscle will oxidize some of the leucine that enters the cell. Also, lysine transport from the blood into the muscle is sluggish. So, the two most prominent EAAs in muscle protein will be selectively limited in terms of availability for incorporation into muscle protein. Consequently, any formulation to stimulate muscle protein synthesis must have higher leucine and lysine concentrations than their respective contributions to muscle protein. As a result of increasing the proportions of leucine and lysine, it is necessary to reduce some or all of the proportions of the other EAAs because if the percent of two goes up, the percent of others must come down so that the total is still 100%. However, the percent contributions of valine and isoleucine should not be reduced on account of increasing the leucine content. When leucine intake increases, not only is leucine oxidation activated, so too is the oxidation of the other two branched chain amino acids.

Special circumstances call for some modifications of the basic formulation. Higher leucine content (35-40% of total EAAs in the supplement) will activate the process of protein synthesis in anabolic resistance, such as aging or cancer. The EAA tryptophan is not important for synthesis of muscle protein, but tryptophan plays an important role as the precursor for the neurotransmitter serotonin. It may be important to provide tryptophan in order to maintain proper balance of neurotransmitters whenever a dose of leucine is given, since both EAAs can compete for the same transporter into the brain.

There are any number of conditions in which a slight modification of the basic formula to stimulate muscle protein synthesis would be appropriate, and as scientists and physicians realize the tremendous potential for specifically-designed formulations of EAAs, more will become available. With regard to the stimulation of muscle protein synthesis, however, years of research have gone into developing formulations based on the principles described in this section. Consequently, when I have referred to EAA supplements I have been referring to a formulation designed to optimally stimulate muscle protein synthesis.

Caloric Equivalents of EAA Supplements

I have addressed in some detail the calories consumed in the context of the protein food sources. The benefits of EAA supplements in this regard are obvious. I showed you the results of studies in which consumption of an EAA supplement containing minimal calories (less than 50 kcal) provides at least three times the stimulation of protein synthesis as any high-quality dietary protein. So, if we consider the case of a 7 g dose between meals to avoid loss of muscle protein, this would be the physiological equivalent of 21 g of high quality protein, with a caloric equivalent of 28 kcal. If we consider a 21 g dose of high quality protein (consider beef), then a total of 147 kcal would be consumed (accounting for both the protein and non-protein component of the beef). In other words, physiologically equivalent dosages of beef and an EAA supplement would differ by five-fold in the total caloric equivalents. Further, keep in mind that the diet-induced thermogenesis resulting from EAA consumption as well as the energy used for the stimulation of protein synthesis both reduce the effective calories of an EAA supplement. The net result is that an EAA supplement has almost no impact on total caloric intake.

The intense effectiveness of EAA supplements and the low caloric equivalent enable you to make up whatever deficit in high quality protein you may have in your basic diet without markedly altering the total caloric intake.

Dosage and Timing of EAA Supplementation

The section on the basic diet referred to the amount of calories as protein. This is reasonable since the caloric intake in the form of protein is a significant part of total caloric intake, and total caloric intake can vary considerably, depending on gender, age, body size, and activity level. The dosage and timing of EAA supplements, on the other hand, are generally referred to in gram amounts. This is because the caloric intake with a pure EAA supplement is insignificant in the context of total caloric intake, and the supplements are generally sold in gram (g) units.

The response to EAA supplements is dose dependent. A dose of as little as 3 grams can stimulate muscle protein synthesis as much as 20 grams of whey protein. Almost 6 grams of muscle protein is produced from consumption of a 3 gram supplement because the perfect balance of EAAs enables the muscle to incorporate all of the EAAs into protein. In addition, the reutilization of NEAAs already in the body contributes to the total amount of protein produced.

While a dosage as small as 3 grams can be effective over time, the amount of muscle protein made from the supplement is limited by the small amount of EAAs consumed. The amount of protein produced in response to EAA intake increases linearly up to a dose of 15 grams of EAAs. Quite simply, a bigger dose will give you a bigger response, up to 15 grams. Beyond that dose, the increase in the amount of protein produced begins to taper off.

The EAAs can be consumed either as powder in capsules or as a beverage, or a combination. It is generally important to use pure EAAs without significant non-protein calories, beyond what is needed for flavoring. The only exception would be a meal replacement based on EAAs but that addresses all nutrient requirements.

Optimally, the EAA supplement should be taken twice a day, between meals or before going to bed. The general idea behind the use of the EAA supplement is to maintain an adequate supply of amino acids throughout the day to support various functions without the interruptions that normally occur when food is not being absorbed. Timing and dosages of EAA supplements are dealt with below in the sections providing specific recommendations for individualized needs.

If you are taking EAA supplements because your regular diet falls short in meeting the recommended intake of high-quality protein, then, in addition to the between-meal doses, you should take supplements with your meals to enhance the physiological effectiveness of the protein intake. The dosage with meals to make up for dietary deficiencies depends on how far short your diet falls of the goal intake of high quality protein, but in the case of a vegetarian diet, this could be up to 15 g of EAAs with each meal to obtain optimal results.

The Physical Activity Plan

The third leg of the EAASE program is physical activity. I distinguish regular physical activity from exercise training, which I address in another section.

No matter the purpose of exercising, the same questions always arise. How much should I exercise and what type of exercise is best? There are very specific guidelines offered by the American College of Sports Medicine (ACSM). ACSM, the largest sports medicine and exercise organization, issued guidelines in 2010: (http://www.acsm.org/about-acsm/media-room/news-releases/2011/08/01/acsm-issues-new-recommendations-on-quantity-and-quality-of-exercise). Those recommendations are consistent with the physical activity guidelines issued by both the American Heart Association and Health and Human Services and are quite specific about the amount of time that should be devoted to physical activity to achieve health benefits. Since these recommendations are based on outcomes related to health, I will present them in total. I will then tell you how the EAASE program relates to these recommendations.

Aerobic Exercise

Aerobic exercise is the type of physical activity that works your heart and lungs for at least 10 minutes, and preferably longer. Walking, jogging, cycling, and elliptical or stairclimbing machines, and aerobic dancing are all examples of aerobic exercise. The initial goal for the EAASE program is to start (or work up to) 30 minutes of aerobic exercise every day. Since some of the training effect can be accrued in increments, the workout can be broken into smaller segments of at least 10 minutes until you are able to work out continuously for 30 minutes. The total amount of exercise and duration should be increased upward until you reach the goals that you set for yourself.

Muscle function will improve with aerobic training. Once you have started training, your long-term goal should be to work out for one solid hour. As a minimum, exercising at 30% of your maximal intensity will yield some benefits. This effort level is low, comparable to a steady walking pace for an untrained person. For comparison, moderate aerobic activity (~50% of maximal intensity) would be a brisk walk, cycling at 10 to 12 miles an hour, or swimming leisurely. Vigorous activity includes jogging or running, cycling fast (at least 12 miles an hour), hiking, cross-country skiing, or swimming moderately hard.

The "talk test" is one way to check your exercise intensity. You're getting moderate aerobic activity if you can talk but can't sing while doing an activity. Another way to gauge exercise intensity is to monitor your heart rate. Moderate aerobic activity is 60% to 70% of your maximum heart rate (220 minus your age). One trick to up the intensity of the workout is to include intervals, brief periods of higher intensity mixed in with lower intensity phases. There is no magic formula here and the more effort you put in, the more benefits you will reap, provided you don't over-extend and injure yourself. The ultimate goal is to be as active as possible while enjoying the activity. This also means that you should find the right mix to avoid risk of injury, overtraining, and obsessive behavior.

ACSM Guidelines for Aerobic Exercise

- Adults should get at least 150 minutes of moderate-intensity exercise per week.
- Exercise recommendations can be met through 30-60 minutes of moderate-intensity exercise (five days per week) or 20-60 minutes of vigorous-intensity exercise (three days per week).
- One continuous session and multiple shorter sessions (of at least 10 minutes) are both acceptable to accumulate the desired amount of daily exercise.

- Gradual progression of exercise time, frequency and intensity is recommended for best adherence and least injury risk.
- People unable to meet these minimums can still benefit from some activity.

Resistance or strength training is the use of resistance to muscular contraction to build strength, anaerobic endurance and size of skeletal muscles. You strengthen and tone your muscles by contracting them against a resisting force. There are two types of resistance training. Isometric resistance involves exerting your muscles against a non-moving object, such as against the floor in a push-up. In this motion, the length of the muscle does not change so there is no contraction of the muscle. Isotonic strength training involves contracting your muscles through a range of motion as in weight lifting.

If you have access to a gym or fitness center, there are many options to build muscles and strength. Weight Lifting can be done with free weights like barbells or on machines (Life Fitness, PowerTec, and Nautilus, to name a few). The advantage of using machines is that the weight is balanced for you and they restrict your body in a fixed movement pattern which will lessen the chance of injury and ensure that specific muscle groups are exercised. If using free weights, it is important to get proper instruction on lifting techniques to avoid injury. Exercises that use your own body weight as resistance are very effective but can be hard at first if you lack sufficient strength. Examples of body-weight exercises include pull-ups, chin-ups, dips, push-ups, crunches and bicycles. Since our bodies adapt to stress relatively quickly, the resistance (amount of weight or number of repetitions) should be increased systematically. There is flexibility in how to approach weight lifting since the cumulative amount of weight lifted is the determinant of the muscle response. This means that if you prefer to lift lighter weights with more repetitions as opposed to fewer lifts with heavier weight, the stress on the muscle is the same as long as the total amount of weight lifted is the same.

Recognize that hitting plateaus is common and you may need to back off on weight increases for a period to move forward. Also, depending on your goals and how often you work out, you may not want to keep increasing the weight loads in your workout. You can maintain your strength and muscle mass, once you have reached the level you desire by repeating your workout two to three times a week. Your muscles need time to recover from weight training so ideally it should be done on alternate days. It is also important to take some time to warm up and cool down after strength training. Combining weight training with EAA supplementation is particularly important to amplify the effects of each.

ACSM Guidelines for Resistance Exercise

- Adults should train each major muscle group two or three days each week using a variety of exercises and equipment.
- Very light or light intensity is best for older persons or previously sedentary adults starting exercise.
- Two to four sets of each exercise will help adults improve strength and power.
- For each exercise, 8-12 repetitions improve strength and power, 10-15 repetitions improve strength in middle-age and older persons starting exercise, and 15-20 repetitions improve muscular endurance.
- Adults should wait at least 48 hours between resistance training sessions.

Adapting the Exercise Guidelines for Your Use

As you can see, the recommended exercise can be fairly rigorous. These workouts were thoughtfully based on the bulk of the scientific literature concerning the workload necessary to achieve physical benefits. However, you may need to adapt them for your own circumstance.

It may take you some time to work up to the amount of different types of exercise recommended by the ACSM. Not everyone can accomplish every aspect of the guidelines right away. Physical capacity may be limiting, and the lack of desire to exercise may be a problem as well. The key to adapting the recommendations for your personal circumstance is to focus on convenient activities that you like to do. Jogging for 30 minutes every day may cause dread for many but taking your dog to the park or beach and running around can allow you to happily accumulate the same number of minutes of aerobic activity.

Setting goals is important if you are going to stick to an exercise program. It is very easy to find excuses and put off your workout if you don't have a goal that you are working towards and a timeframe in which to achieve the goal. The goal must be manageable and realistic in order to avoid failure and discouragement. For example, if you've never run more than a mile, it might be overly ambitious to make running a marathon your goal. It's best to set short-term and long-term goals. Another motivational technique is to join a sports club and engage in an activity like softball, golf, basketball, soccer, or any of the multitude of activities available in most communities. It is possible to meet the goals of the ACSM guidelines with a variety of activities.

Don't Sit Too Much!

The exercise guidelines are focused on workouts. It is quite common that if you do a workout, you feel like the hay is in the barn for the day and there is no need to get out of a chair for the rest of the day. This is particularly true if you have an office job. However, recent evidence shows that you can lose much of the benefit of exercise training if you then sit for the rest of the day. For example, exercise can improve your lipid profile in the blood, but if you spend an excessive amount of time sitting for the rest of the day, you can undo the beneficial effect of the exercise. It is important that you get up from your desk or TV and walk around; don't take the elevator, use the stairs, etc. There are plenty of ways to avoid the problems stemming from too much sitting.

EAA Supplements and Exercise

There are cardiovascular and metabolic benefits of both aerobic and resistance exercise. The benefits of the exercise can be amplified by coordinating the timing of your EAA supplement consumption. The exercise primes both the heart and skeletal muscle to respond to an increased availability of EAAs.

In the case of aerobic exercise, you should take the EAAs after exercise. Taking them before exercise will reduce their efficiency, since a high proportion will be oxidized during the exercise.

When performing resistance exercise you will get the most benefit from your EAA supplement if you take it 30 minutes before exercise. In order to fully capitalize on the "priming" of the synthetic machinery in muscle, you should take a second dose of EAAs within the first hour after completion of exercise. With this approach, the magnitude of the stimulation of muscle protein turnover will be much greater than achieved with either the exercise or supplements alone. You can also benefit from taking EAAs during a resistance workout.

How Long Do I Need to Stick to the EAASE Program, and What Can I Expect?

The EAASE program is meant as a lifestyle program. You should follow the basic guidelines for the rest of your life. You will reap the benefits as long as you follow the program. The benefits of the program will be lost if you stop following the recommendations.

Following the EAASE program will give you more energy to do the activities you enjoy. Your metabolic health will improve, including insulin sensitivity, blood pressure and blood lipids. You will gradually improve your body composition, losing fat and gaining muscle mass. This will be reflected in the way you feel, and the way your clothes fit. You will feel stronger.

The beneficial changes will take some time to achieve. Nutrition and exercise do not cause immediate results. You need to commit to at least 6 weeks of adhering to the program before judging if you are benefitting in the expected way.

Are There Possible Adverse Effects of the EAASE Program?

The program is designed for minimal risk. The dietary recommendations for high quality protein are well within the limits of the Acceptable Macronutrient Distribution Range of the National Academy of Sciences. The exercise recommendations are within the guidelines of the American College of Sports Medicine. The essential amino acids in EAA supplements are all Generally Regarded as Safe (GRAS) by the FDA and have no adverse effects when taken as EAA supplements (i.e., all the EAAs taken together).

Essentials

- The EAASE program targets the muscle, liver, heart and brain. The main focus for healthy young to middle-aged individuals is muscle protein synthesis.
- The EAASE Program consists of a healthy regular diet, an appropriate EAA supplement, and exercise.
- The crucial aspect of the diet in the EAASE program is the percentage of total caloric intake you consume as protein. In general, the target is to consume 25% of your calories as high quality protein.
- You can figure out how much dietary protein you should eat by first estimating your caloric requirement and multiplying that value by the desired fraction of caloric intake as high quality protein.
- You can estimate your dietary caloric intake by keeping dietary records, or estimating your dietary caloric requirement from the estimation of daily energy expenditure. The basal energy expenditure is calculated using the Harris-Benedict equation. That value is multiplied by an activity factor to determine total energy requirement.
- Total energy requirement is multiplied by the fraction of calories as protein (0.25 or more depending upon your goal and preference) to determine how many calories as protein you should eat.
- The calories as protein can be converted to ounces of protein food sources using the USDA Nutrient Data Base. Examples are provided, along with how to calculate the kcal per ounce of protein as well as the total kcal per ounce protein food source.
- Comprehensive guidelines for exercise are provided by the American College of Sports Medicine (www.acsm.org).
- You should adapt the exercise program to activities that you enjoy and that you will do regularly into the foreseeable future.

- EAA supplements are taken between meals to stop the net loss of muscle protein that occurs between meals, and to make up for inadequate EAA intake in the regular diet. EAA supplements are particularly important if you eat a vegetarian diet.
- An EAA supplement in conjunction with exercise will amplify the beneficial effects of the exercise, and the exercise will amplify the beneficial effects of the EAA supplement.
- General Guidelines for the basic EAASE program.
  o Basic diet: 25% of caloric intake as high quality protein.
  o Two doses of 7 g (for the basic program) each of EAAs taken between meals.
  o Resistance exercise twice per week, aerobic exercise 4-5 times per week.
    ▪ Resistance: 15 g dose of EAAs before and after workout.
    ▪ Aerobic: 15 g dose of EAAs after workout.

The EAASE Program for Specific Circumstances

The general principles of the EAASE program discussed above apply to everyone. Specific conditions may call for some fine-tuning of its components based on the physiological responses to the condition, and your personal goals.

The EAASE Program for Maintaining Muscle Mass and Function in Aging.

While it is impossible to entirely stop the process of aging, it is definitely possible to slow the progression of muscle loss. In most cases, sarcopenia is a preventable condition. The EAASE program is proven to improve both strength and muscle mass. It is preferable to start this program before sarcopenia is established, but even sarcopenic individuals can benefit from the EAASE program. It is important to realize that there is no fountain of youth, but the changes in diet, consumption of EAAs, and regular exercise as outlined in the EAASE program can curtail the rate of decline in muscle strength and mass that comes with aging.

The Basic Diet

The principles of the EAASE program apply to your everyday diet regardless of your age. The key is to eat at least 25% of your calories in the form of high quality protein. This percentage translates to about 500 kcal of high quality protein for a person over 65 years of age. The examples based on the data shown previously in Table 2 should help you to figure out what this recommendation translates to in terms of protein food sources. The remainder of the diet is flexible and should include a variety of fruits and vegetables as well as whatever special treats you might enjoy.

The principles of the basic diet apply regardless of age, with one little bonus for older people. As you get older, your ideal body weight (as defined by body mass index) increases. It is inevitable that you will pass through some health challenges as you age, and having a little extra weight gives you a cushion that can help in these circumstances. Consequently, you don't need to worry as much about putting on a few pounds as you did when you were younger. (Note: this may be the best thing about getting old!). It is much better to be sure you eat enough than to think you are doing something good for yourself by eating lightly to lose some weight. Of course, you cannot take this to an extreme, as obesity is the major factor limiting mobility in older people.

EAA Supplements

EAA supplements can benefit everyone (thus the acronym EAASE). EAA supplements are a particularly important part of dietary intake in older people. With aging a number of factors can conspire to result in decreased consumption of high quality proteins. As a result, the amount of EAAs consumed is likely to be reduced. Even if you eat 25% of caloric intake as high quality protein, your EAA intake has probably fallen below the level of intake when you were younger, since you are probably eating less total calories. Nonetheless, the EAASE program does not advocate increasing the consumption of more dietary protein as a percent of caloric intake than for younger people for several reasons. First, dramatic changes in your regular dietary pattern are difficult to stick with and can be stressful because of the time, effort, and potential cost involved in changing your routine. Also, anabolic resistance that accompanies aging reduces the effectiveness of dietary protein. It is more beneficial to increase your consumption of EAAs by incorporating EAA supplements in your overall dietary pattern.

An EAA supplement can be formulated to overcome anabolic resistance, and thus be much more effective than natural protein food sources in terms of stimulating muscle protein synthesis. Further, EAAs present less of a burden to the liver and kidneys than intact protein. An EAA supplement designed for anabolic resistance not only stimulates muscle protein synthesis, but also causes an increased recycling of NEAAs back into protein. In contrast, ingested dietary proteins add more NEAAs into circulation. Surplus NEAAs are metabolized by the liver and ultimately produce urea and ammonia which are excreted in urine by the kidney. Reutilizing NEAAs in circulation by providing only EAAs means less work for the liver and the kidneys. The kidneys benefit since they do not have to excrete extra urea and ammonia in the urine.

The optimal amount of a balanced EAA supplement for older individuals is 15 grams taken twice per day between meals. This dosage will elicit the maximal stimulatory effect on protein synthesis and thus gain in muscle mass over time. Smaller and less frequent doses are also effective in stimulating muscle protein synthesis, but the effectiveness is reduced in proportion to the reduction in dose. A dose as small as 3 grams has the equivalent effect of as much as 20 grams of high quality protein on stimulating muscle protein synthesis. The dose of EAA you choose to use will depend on a number of factors. If you are eating a diet relatively deficient in EAAs, then larger doses of an EAA supplement are essential. If you are exercising, the timing of the ingestion of the EAA supplement should be coordinated with the exercise, as described below. The EAAs should be taken in the free form with minimal mixing with other nutrients. Powder mixed into a beverage is the most convenient, but capsules can be an effective way to consume part of your dose as well.

Exercise

Exercise is a key component of the EAASE program. You are no doubt aware that regular exercise can play a pivotal role in maintaining muscle mass and function, and can be the key to a happy and productive retirement.

The unique aspect of the EAASE program is that EAA supplements are used to amplify the beneficial effects of exercise.

Resistance exercise is the most effective way to maintain muscle mass and strength. Don't think you are too old to do resistance exercise; individuals in their 90's have improved their muscle strength and function as a result of a resistance exercise program. Detailed instructions are not necessary, as studies have shown that the exact nature of the exercises make much less difference than the total amount of weight lifted. For example, 3 sets of 10 repetitions lifting 20 lbs will give you the same result as 3 sets of 4 repetitions lifting 50 lbs. Injuries are less likely to result with multiple repetitions using lighter weights. It doesn't really matter exactly what exercises you do, as long as you exercise a variety of muscles and lift enough weight to feel the effort.

The important thing to remember about resistance exercise is that you are priming your muscle to respond to the anabolic effect of EAAs. Resistance exercise cannot increase muscle protein synthesis in a significant way without substrates (i.e., EAAs) from which to make the protein. If you take EAAs 30 minutes before working out, you prevent the breakdown of muscle protein that would otherwise occur during exercise. Taking another dose of EAAs after the workout will amplify the exercise effect on muscle protein synthesis, with the net being a greater increase in both mass and function than would occur in response to either exercise or EAAs alone.

There is also a beneficial interaction between EAAs and aerobic exercise. In the case of aerobic exercise, the EAAs should be taken after exercise, since a significant portion of the EAAs taken before exercise will be oxidized during the exercise.

The exercise component of the EAASE program is intentionally flexible. The only absolute in the program is that you take EAAs before and after resistance exercise and after aerobic exercise. A description of specific exercises is left vague because there is a huge range in capabilities of older individuals and personal preferences. Rather than give you a specific exercise prescription, I would like to share with you some general perspectives about exercise.

If you are an older individual reading this book you probably fall into one of two categories, either you have not done much physical activity for years, or you still workout and/or participate in active sports such as golf or tennis or even jogging.

If you haven't done any kind of exercise for years, you will probably benefit from some help from a certified exercise trainer to develop a program specifically designed for your capabilities and goals. Regardless of the program, you will have to learn how to push yourself again. You are in the enviable position that you will see rapid improvement as you begin to train, whatever the exercise you choose. The improvement will be especially dramatic if you couple your exercise with EAA supplements. Your improvement will inspire you to stay with whatever program you have laid out for yourself. However, be aware that at some point you will plateau in your progress. When you hit a plateau, you will need to push harder to keep improving. Don't baby yourself! You are capable of more than you realize. The key to success is consistency. You have to make your exercise time an un-negotiable time of the day. Getting in a rigid schedule and adhering to it is the surest way to get the consistency that you need.

If you have exercised all your life, your perspective will be quite different than if you are starting up a program after years of sedentary life style. Although you have the tremendous advantage that you are probably in much better shape than the average person

244

your age, you still face challenges. The challenges are part physical and part psychological, and the two aspects may merge together indistinguishably. I can relate some of my experiences in this regard, as I fall into this group and have talked with many former athletes in the same situation as myself.

When I was young, my athletic focus was basketball, but after that phase was finished, I took up distance running seriously. Although not a world class runner, I nonetheless embraced the challenge of setting both short-term and long-term goals and training hard to try to reach those goals. I trained and raced steadily from the time I was 25 years old until last year at 69 when I had my hip replaced. Being a scientist, I approached training for marathons methodically. I carefully recorded every workout in detail, with the distance, time, etc. I did interval workouts twice per week and recorded every split of every interval.

As I got older, I faced challenges that all of my friends who ran also faced. Of course, there were the usual injuries. They not only became more frequent as I got older, but it took longer to recover. But most discouragingly, I inevitably got progressively slower. I was 65 when I last trained for a full marathon. I was still trying to do the same program as when I was younger, but with drastically less success. I was running quarter-mile intervals at a considerably slower pace than I could maintain for an entire 26 mile marathon when I was younger. Intellectually, I understood that the days of 65-second quarter mile intervals were long in the rear view mirror, but psychologically, it was much harder to accept. I would look at the workouts in my running log that I used to do and feel overwhelmingly discouraged at the decline in my ability. I could understand why almost everyone I knew from years of running had given it up.

At some point, I assessed things and decided that I would rather keep running at a slower pace and within my realistic capabilities than to quit it altogether. I started a new running log, and put the old ones away and forgot about what I used to do. I wish I could say that, all of a sudden I saw the light and loved running again, but it doesn't really work that way. I still get frustrated when jogging and someone breezes by me like I'm standing still. Nonetheless, I have made enough peace with my current abilities that I keep plugging away every day. I now take naps after good workouts, as I recognize I don't recover very fast anymore. I certainly use more ibuprofen than I used to. I never question why I am still working out - it's just what I do.

The lesson from my personal story is that the important thing as you get older is to keep doing whatever activity or sport that you like to do. You have to get past the dismay that you need to play from the forward tees on the golf course when you used to play from the tips, or that you can only play doubles in tennis now. The benefits of participation in activities you enjoy will trump any of the negative aspects. The social aspect of joining workout classes in the gym or a group to play golf with regularly is an important step in the adjustment to retirement. You just need to let go of what you used to do, and be happy with what you can do now.

How will You Know the EAASE Program is Working?

After about a month to six weeks of committing to the diet and exercise recommendations, you will start to feel the effects. You will feel more energy to engage in the activities you enjoy, and recover much faster. You won't necessarily lose weight (muscle weighs more than fat), but your clothes will start fitting better. You will feel more fit.

Essentials

- The EAASE program for maintaining muscle mass and function in aging:
    - The basic diet contains approximately 25% of calories as high quality protein.
    - Regular exercise. Preferably, resistance exercise twice per week and aerobic exercise four days a week. Do activities you like!
    - EAA supplement (up to 15 g) (with a high proportion of leucine) is taken twice per day:
        - Between meals if you are not exercising
        - Before and after resistance exercise
        - After aerobic exercise

The EAASE Program for Athletic Training

There is a wide range of competitive sports, and body types that excel in the different sports vary accordingly. Even in the same sport different positions call for distinct body types. Think about the body type of football players- a wide receiver might weigh as much as 200 pound less than an offensive guard. Training and nutritional goals differ accordingly. Fortunately, the EAASE program can easily be adapted to whatever the goal might be. This flexibility exists because the program is based on basic principles of nutrition and muscle protein metabolism rather than sport-specific tips.

Endurance Sports

Endurance sports include running, swimming, cycling, rowing, etc. These activities are often called aerobic sports, since much of the training is done aerobically. Since competitive racing almost always has anaerobic components, both in competition as well as training (think intervals), it is more appropriate to refer to the combination of aerobic and anaerobic training as endurance sports. Because training is so sport-specific, I will not discuss the workouts, but rather focus on how the use of EAA supplements can amplify the training effects of your workouts, as well as the regular diet for endurance sports.

The EAASE program has an important role in training for endurance sports. There are two principle ways in which muscle adapts during training, 1) the muscle fibers contract more effectively, 2) the muscle mitochondria increase in number and efficiency in producing energy. An increase in protein turnover is the metabolic basis for all of these physiological adaptations that enable improved performance. Increased protein turnover enables muscle to function more efficiently because fibers that are not functioning well are broken down and replaced by new fibers that have superior contraction characteristics.

The increase in mitochondria with endurance training occurs because they divide more rapidly. Once the mitochondria divide, the proteins in the mitochondria (called enzymes) must be produced at an increased rate to enable the chemical reactions that produce energy to proceed.

Interaction of EAA Supplements and Training

Both training and EAAs promote all of the adaptations of muscle protein metabolism described above. Importantly, when training and EAAs are combined, the effects are greater than the sum of the individual effects of training and EAAs. Further, the benefits of EAAs can be obtained with minimal caloric intake. This is important for most endurance athletes, as extra body

250

weight is generally a liability. It is important to consume 15 g of EAAs immediately following each workout to maximize the training effect. If you are doing two workouts per day, you will find that the EAA supplement after the first workout speeds recovery for the second workout. The EAAs also help recovery from day to day. If you are doing only one workout per day, then the second dose should be taken before bed so that muscle protein turnover will remain accelerated throughout the night.

Following the recommended program for EAA supplements contributes a mere 120 calories to overall energy intake. Furthermore, since EAA intake stimulates metabolic rate (due to the caloric requirement of increased protein turnover), the effective amount of calories is even less. EAA supplements are the most effective way to amplify your muscle adaptations to training without gaining weight.

The Basic Diet

The EAASE program involves recommendations for your basic diet. As with all circumstances, the principle starting point in the optimal diet for endurance exercise is eating high quality protein. This will help you to maintain the high rate of protein turnover necessary for adaptation of your muscle to the stress of training and competing. The target of 25% of calories as high quality protein is well suited for most recreational athletes. However, if you are seriously training for an endurance sport, you are expending a large amount of energy. Consuming 25% of your caloric intake as high quality protein, in this case, is probably not a reasonable goal. For example, a caloric intake of 5,000 kcal per day or more may be needed to stay in energy balance if you are training twice per day. If you strive to eat 25% of this large number of calories as protein, you would have to consume more than 300 g of protein per day. This amount of protein may be beneficial in some circumstances. For example, power athletes routinely eat this much protein in order to gain muscle mass. However, as an endurance athlete your goal is not to gain muscle mass. Further, the non-protein calories associated with 300 g of high-quality protein could present problems. Depending upon the food source, as much as 500 g of dietary fat may accompany the protein calories if you rely on animal-based protein. Because of the high energy density of fat as compared to carbohydrate, that much fat would virtually meet your total caloric requirements without room in your diet for any carbohydrates. Carbohydrate intake is essential in endurance training to restore your glycogen stores that have been depleted by your workouts.

Endurance training is the one circumstance that the EAASE program involves deriving a significant part of your dietary protein from plant-based food sources. There are two reasons for highly trained athletes to rely to some extent on plant-based proteins. First, total caloric requirement is so high that even with lower quality plant-based proteins making up a significant portion of the daily protein intake, you will still be getting an abundant amount of EAAs. Second, you can select plant-based protein food sources in which the non-protein calories are carbohydrate.

When you assess the protein content of your regular diet, you may find that you are well below the goal of 25% of calories as protein. The most efficient way to make up the difference between your goal and actual intake is to increase the dosage and number of EAA supplements, as well as adding protein supplements such as whey protein isolate. In this way, you can meet your dietary EAA goals while leaving enough flexibility in the remainder of your dietary pattern for fruit, vegetables and starches that will provide micronutrients as well as replete muscle glycogen.

Power Sports

As with endurance sports, there is a wide variety of power sports, each with their own training regimen. The EAASE program is meant as an adjunct that will make your training more effective. As in the case of training for endurance sports, you undoubtedly have your own training regimen to fulfill the exercise component of the EAASE program.

Interaction of EAA Supplements and Training

The research documenting the optimal use of EAA supplements with weight training is extensive. Consuming 15 grams of EAAs 30 min before starting your workout will elevate the blood EAA concentrations throughout your workout and stop the breakdown of muscle protein that would otherwise occur. 15 grams of EAAs achieves a greater response on muscle protein synthesis than 40 grams of whey protein, without creating the fullness that can hinder a workout. When you complete your workout, consume another 15 grams of EAAs. For a maximal anabolic response, consume another 15 grams of EAAs before bed time, and set your alarm to have a final dose at about 4 a.m. if you are really committed to maximizing the gain in muscle. The 4 a.m. dose will limit the breakdown in muscle protein that otherwise occurs overnight when you are not absorbing protein. This supplementation pattern will turn what is normally a catabolic state during the night time in which you are losing muscle into an anabolic state in which you gain muscle.

The sum of these doses totals 60 grams/day. This amount of EAAs is needed to drive protein synthesis past what may be your normal genetic limitation.

The Basic Diet

Power sports require getting big. We all have genetic limitations, and to be big enough to play an interior lineman in football or throw the shot competitively often will stress a body to its absolute genetic limitations. Protein is the key dietary component of the basic diet. It will increase your muscle mass. You should set a goal of eating approximately 30% of your caloric intake as high quality protein. Again, as with the example given above, eating this amount of high-quality protein food sources may present problems in terms of lack of flexibility of non-protein calories, EAA supplements will play a vital role in helping you to meet your dietary goal for EAA intake.

While the focus of your basic diet should be high quality protein, you must remember that energy substrates (carbohydrates and fat) are important too. As an example, in a tightly controlled study, subjects drank the same amount of protein in the form of milk. In one case, it was skim milk, and in the other case whole milk. The stimulation of muscle protein synthesis was greater with the whole milk. Under these study conditions, the additional calories provided by the fat in the whole milk helped to fuel the muscle building.

You must be in positive energy balance to gain a significant amount of muscle mass. Carbohydrate is of less importance for resistance training than endurance training, but you should eat enough fruit and vegetables to meet the RDAs for micronutrients. Also, carbohydrate intake will stimulate insulin release, and insulin is an anabolic hormone that will increase the amount of muscle protein made from your EAA intake. Fat intake will also amplify the anabolic effect of EAAs, and therefore you can eat animal-based high-quality protein foods without worrying about eating too much fat.

The key with regard to your basic diet is that the more you eat, the bigger you will get. If you do this while lifting heavy weights and consuming EAA supplements as recommended, a significant part of the weight gain will be muscle. You will also gain fat with this dietary approach, so you need to carefully monitor your body composition to be sure that the extra fat you put on does not counteract the benefits of the muscle gain. In a sport like power lifting, that is not likely to be the case, but in a sport like throwing the shot in which speed and agility are factors, you must reach a balance between muscle and fat gains.

Essentials

- The EAASE program for endurance training:
  - The basic diet aims for 25% of calories as protein. A combination of animal- and plant-based protein sources are recommended to include sufficient carbohydrate intake. Protein supplements may be required to achieve the protein goal while consuming enough carbohydrates to replete muscle glycogen after workouts.
  - Consume 15 grams of EAAs immediately after your workout. If you are doing two workouts a day, then consume the EAA supplements after each workout. If you are doing one workout per day, consume the second 15 gram dose of EAAs before bed.
- The EAASE program for power sports:
  - The regular diet: aim for 30% of calories as high-quality protein, enough calories as fat and carbohydrate to be in positive energy balance.
  - EAA supplements (15 gram doses) 30 minutes before and immediately after workout.
  - EAA supplements (15 grams) before bed and at 4 a.m.

The EAASE Program for Weight Loss

The Underlying Principle

Ultimately, all weight-loss programs are about creating a negative energy balance, meaning that the amount of energy you consume over the day is less than the amount of energy you expend. Calories are the unit of energy, so negative energy balance means that caloric intake is less than caloric expenditure. EAASE is unique among the myriad of weight loss programs in that it is focused not only on weight loss, but the quality of the weight loss in terms of body composition.

The underlying principle of the EAASE program for weight loss is that muscle mass should be preserved, meaning that lost weight should be entirely in the form of fat. Preserving muscle mass during weight loss is a challenge because preservation of muscle mass is not only a function of dietary protein intake, but also total caloric intake. Reduction of caloric intake potentially affects muscle mass negatively in two ways. First, if you do not change the composition of the diet, reducing your caloric intake to half your normal level will also cut the amount of protein intake in half. Expressed differently, just to maintain the same amount of dietary protein intake that you normally eat, you will have to double the percent of calories eaten as protein. For example, if you are following the general EAASE guidelines and consume 25% of your calories as protein, to maintain the level of protein in your diet constant during weight loss, protein will have to comprise 50% of your caloric intake. Given that most protein foods provide at least half of their calories as carbohydrate and/or fat, the entire diet may have to be composed of foods from the protein food group.

The second aspect of negative energy balance is that maintaining the rate of muscle protein synthesis is much harder when calories are cut. Think back to the example of whole milk stimulating muscle building more than lower calorie fat free milk. It has been known for more than 100 years that the level of protein intake needed to maintain a balance between protein synthesis and breakdown is influenced by the amount of energy intake which fuels the energy cost of protein synthesis.

Muscle can only be preserved during caloric restriction weight loss if an adequate amount of EAAS are available to stimulate muscle protein synthesis sufficiently to maintain muscle mass in the circumstance of a negative energy balance. Basing your dietary regimen on the use of free EAAs is the most effective and practical approach to accomplishing this goal.

The EAASE program not only aims to maintain muscle mass, but to maintain a high rate of muscle protein turnover (i.e., synthesis and breakdown). The process of muscle protein turnover uses energy, and therefore works in favor of weight loss. A high rate of muscle protein turnover also improves the function of individual muscle fibers, and therefore benefits muscular function.

Caloric Restriction Weight Loss with EAAs

The EAASE strategy for weight loss relies on EAA-enhanced meal substitutes to simplify the weight-loss process. Fifteen grams of free EAA are included with each meal substitute. The free EAAs will overcome the limitations of caloric restriction on muscle protein synthesis. This can be accomplished by using an EAA-based meal replacement (if available), or by adding the free EAAs to a high-protein meal replacement. The EAA-enriched meal substitute can either be used for the entire diet or to substitute for an individual meal.

The goal of the diet is to consume a bout 1,200 kcal/day. This level of calorie intake results in clinically-significant weight loss for most people. It is most convenient to rely heavily on meal substitutes. For example, conventional meal substitutes such as Optifast or Bariatric Advantage have approximately 160 -170 kcal. If 15 g of EAAs are taken with each meal substitute, that would add an additional 60 kcal per meal. Six doses of the combination of meal substitutes plus free EAAs would provide approximately 1,200 kcal. A multivitamin should be taken to ensure that no deficiencies result from the reduced nutrient intake.

Adherence to a diet based entirely on meal substitutes providing about 1,200 kcal per day will result in approximately 12-15 pounds of weight loss in three months. The free amino acids will stimulate muscle protein turnover, thereby raising metabolic rate and contributing to weight loss. The advantage to this approach is that it takes food choices and serving sizes out of the equation. Most importantly, fat will be virtually the entire source of weight loss.

The diet described above could be called a "total immersion" approach. Many find it possible to stick to this kind of approach for a limited number of months. The greatest success with this approach is usually with closely supervised programs. However, it is not a realistic approach for long-term. An alternative approach is to use a low-calorie diet that supplies about 1,200 kcal, and supplement that with two doses per day of 15 gm of EAAs. The EAA supplementation will overcome the inherent limitation of a regular diet containing only 1,200 kcal per day with respect to maintaining muscle mass, no matter how "high protein" the diet may be. This approach will preserve more muscle than a diet relying entirely on food sources.

In case you want to use the approach of eating a low-calorie diet of regular food, supplemented with free EAAs, it may be most convenient to use a food service that provides pre-made meals that add up to the specified number of calories per day. If that is not appealing or financially possible, it is possible to compose your own diet each day, but you should be forewarned that adherence to a diet relying entirely on your own choice of food can be challenging. Certain programs will provide sample meal plans with specific food choices.

Regardless of the approach to reducing total caloric intake, the diet should be supplemented with at least 2 x 15 g EAA or more to preserve muscle mass without adding substantively to caloric intake.

The Role of Exercise in Weight Loss

Exercise alone is generally ineffective in causing a significant amount of weight loss. For example, walking a mile will burn about 120 kcal. To lose significant weight requires a negative energy balance of about 1,200 kcal per day (meaning that you eat about 1,200 kcal less than you expend). Therefore, you would need to walk about 10 miles per day (and not change your food intake) to get the same energy deficit as caloric restriction. The fact that the caloric expenditure of the exercise generally stimulates the appetite makes it even more difficult to lose weight by exercising without reducing dietary intake.

While relying on increased activity of even organized exercise to lose weight is not likely to be effective by itself, exercise is extremely beneficial in combination with caloric restriction, particularly to preserve muscle. Resistance exercise in particular can help to maintain the muscle mass during weight loss. This synergy is particularly true with the EAASE plan, as the combination of EAAs and resistance exercise will stimulate muscle protein synthesis more than the sum of their individual effects. Aerobic exercise will also be beneficial. Not only will you burn more calories by doing aerobic exercise, but muscle mass will also be retained more effectively. A dietary supplement of 15 g EAAs should be taken after exercise.

Bariatric Surgery

Bariatric surgery has become an important alternative to traditional weight loss methods for a significant number of obese individuals. Interestingly, the surgery seems to have unique metabolic benefits over traditional caloric restriction weight loss in obese individuals. On the negative side, loss of muscle mass can be dramatic as weight is rapidly decreased. This undesirable effect, in part, reflects an impaired ability to digest intact protein effectively. In addition, patients that go through any surgical procedure may develop anabolic resistance, meaning that intact protein loses its normal effectiveness in stimulating muscle protein synthesis.

While the specifics of the EAASE program don't differ in regard to weight loss after bariatric surgery as described above, the rationale is even stronger for the use of EAAs after bariatric surgery. Free EAAs will be extensively digested and absorbed even after bariatric surgery, meaning that their effect on muscle protein turnover will be fully retained. The fact that free EAAs can be formulated to overcome anabolic resistance is another potential advantage of relying on EAA-based nutrition following bariatric surgery.

The exercise component of the EAASE program applies equally to individuals recovering from bariatric surgery.

Maintenance

The term "yo-yo dieting" is familiar to anyone who has had an ongoing problem with weight management. Once the weight is lost, you return to your normal diet, and then the weight goes back on. It is hard not to reward yourself for all the effort it took to lose the weight, so it is not uncommon for the weight to return or even exceed the previous weight loss. Yo-yo dieting over a period of years eventually leads to sarcopenic obesity in older age. Each time you lose weight, you lose both muscle and fat, and when weight is regained, it is predominantly as fat. Repeating this cycle many times gradually erodes your muscle mass, so by the time you are older, you have the same excess body weight to move around with a depleted muscle mass to try to stay mobile.

The EAASE program minimizes the muscle loss when dieting. When you reach your weight loss goal, the program does not leave you high and dry. EAASE offers a weight maintenance strategy. The cornerstone of the weight maintenance program is to consume one meal substitute (including 15 g EAAs) for either breakfast or lunch. This substitution will reduce your daily caloric intake while maintaining a high rate of muscle protein turnover.

Regular exercise is a mandatory aspect of the weight maintenance program. The same rules apply regarding the interaction of EAAs and exercise. If you are doing resistance exercise, take 15 grams of EAAs before and after exercise; if you are doing aerobic exercise, consume 15 grams after exercise. Smaller doses can also be effective, but the magnitude of the beneficial effect is directly related to the amount of EAAs consumed (up to 15 g).

The maintenance program will maintain a high rate of muscle protein turnover, thereby maintaining both muscle mass as well as function. The stimulation of muscle protein synthesis will increase energy expenditure, thereby favorably impacting energy balance.

The EAASE program for weight loss:

- Caloric restriction weight loss
  - 6 x 150 kcal/day dose of meal replacement, including 15 grams EAAs (150 kcal meal replacement + 60 kcal (15 g) EAAs).
  - Daily multi-vitamin.
  - Resistance exercise twice per week, aerobic exercise 4-5 times per week. One of the doses of meal replacement + EAAs should be taken shortly after exercise.
- Maintenance
  - One meal replacement + 15 grams EAAs (150 kcal + 60kcal) as substitute for either breakfast or lunch.
  - Resistance exercise twice per week, aerobic exercise 4-5 times per week. 15 grams of EAAs after aerobic exercise, 15 grams EAAs before and after resistance exercise.

Alternatively, if you are using one of the popular high-protein diets, then consume 15 grams EAA supplement twice per day between meals. The same approach to EAA supplementation in relation to exercise as described above applies.

The EAASE Program for Serious Illness, Injury, and Surgery

Catabolic states involve a rapid loss of muscle mass and include a wide variety of conditions that have in common a rapid loss of muscle mass. Examples of catabolic states include major surgery or trauma, serious chronic diseases like cancer and heart failure, or acute illnesses such as pneumonia. Even a serious case of the flu creates a catabolic state. The primary feature of a catabolic state is the loss of muscle mass at a rate much faster than would occur as a result of decreased dietary protein intake alone.

There are two components of the catabolic state, changes in muscle metabolism that are part of the *stress response*, and a decreased appetite.

The Severe Catabolic State

Many catabolic states involve hospitalization during the most severe stage, perhaps even in the intensive care unit. Nutrition in a severe catabolic state is problematic because the normal anabolic response to protein intake is diminished (anabolic resistance), glucose metabolism is altered significantly (insulin resistance and fat accumulation in the liver), and the fatty acid levels in the blood are elevated. The debilitative effects of bed rest are often superimposed on the stress response in the acutely severe stage of the stress response. In this state, nutrition is generally under the care of a physician. Providing EAAs is a primary goal, as even with anabolic resistance, EAAs can effectively slow down the loss of muscle. Nonetheless, the acutely severe phase of the stress response is not addressed as part of the EAASE program because I do not want to interfere with medical treatment in any way.

Recovery from a Catabolic State

You have probably heard people speak of their ordeal with serious illness or major surgery by saying that the only good part was losing some excess weight, and now they want to keep the weight off. This is such a common response that you may have actually said it yourself, even if after just a bout with the flu or a stomach bug. The problem with this perspective is that the stress response specifically targets muscle loss. Although some fat is lost as well, a significant portion of your weight loss was muscle. Further, you are very likely to regain the weight that you lost in one way or another. The key is to restore your lost muscle mass and not unfavorably affect body composition by regaining your body weight as fat.

The Stress Response Persists after Recovery from the Acute Phase

Even though you have recovered from the most serious part of your illness or injury, the stress response does not instantly turn off. Some aspects of the stress response may persist for a year or more after the acute phase. Consequently, even though you may feel that you have basically recovered, your nutrition must still be geared to the anabolic resistance you suffered in the acute phase. The EAASE plan is ideally suited to enable you to regain your muscle mass in the recovery phase after serious illness or injury, as it favors a preferential gain of muscle as compared to fat.

The Basic Diet

Consuming 25-30% of the calories in your diet as high quality protein will favor gain of muscle as opposed to fat. Initially the anabolic resistance will limit the effectiveness of the dietary protein, but as you improve to full recovery the dietary protein will become more effective. You will benefit by consuming a rather high percentage of your calories as a component of high-quality foods, particularly with the consumption of animal proteins. This recommendation is by design. It may be that as much as 45-50% of your calories are initially in the form of fat. The resistance to the action of insulin persists after the acute phase, and this makes carbohydrate less effective as an energy substrate. It is more likely that the carbohydrate will be converted to fat and stored in the liver. It is therefore reasonable to limit carbohydrate to 20-30% of your caloric intake.

As you regain your muscle mass and approach complete recovery, your basic diet should evolve towards one of the diet options that suits your individual needs and preferences.

Exercise

Exercise is always important in relation to muscle mass and function, and never more so than in recovery from a catabolic state. Exercise is the best way to reverse muscle loss and regain normal function. However, depending on your particular situation, it may be difficult to follow the general guidelines of the American College of Sports Medicine. It may be necessary to go to a physical therapist initially, followed by an experienced trainer, to formulate the best plan for recovery exercises. The general guideline of resistance exercise twice per week and aerobic exercise 5 times per week is appropriate, with the understanding that the level of intensity can be quite limited at first.

I can recount many personal stories related to recovering physical function after surgery. For example, after my hip replacement I was given a set of exercises that would seem pretty lame to someone who didn't just have their hip replaced. I was instructed to do the exercises 5 times per day, which was quite time consuming, but since I had nothing else to do, I stuck with the simple exercises. The physical therapist quickly had me progress to more difficult exercises, and within a few weeks, I was up to where you could call it a "workout". Even then, the extent of debilitation after the surgery was discouraging. The problem was not just the hip, but the feeling of total exhaustion after what, to me, should have been easy workouts. I really didn't feel like doing the exercises, particularly the day after surgery. I have no doubt that being guided through the step of physical recovery by an experienced physical therapist was vital for my rapid recovery. Nonetheless, after a few weeks, I began to feel like I would never get back to where I wanted to be. From experience, though, I knew that there was no substitute for persistence, and the belief that if you persevere, things eventually get better. My energy and strength did come around for me, as it will for you if you fully commit to the program.

EAA Supplements

EAA supplements play a key role in recovery from catabolic stress. The mixture should be formulated to overcome anabolic resistance, with high leucine content. The usage pattern of EAA supplements should target an increase in muscle mass and function. Supplements should be taken between meals to avoid the loss of muscle that normally occurs in the absence of the absorption of dietary protein. As you regain strength, you will want to start coordinating the timing of your supplement intake with your exercise routine as described above. However, in the recovery stage you will be doing very light activity many times a day. With this pattern of activity, it will be just as effective to take the supplements between meals as to try to coordinate with the light exercises you will be doing. Regardless of how light the exercise is, it is in fact activating the muscle to begin the process of restoration to full strength.

Essentials

The EAASE Program for catabolic states:

- Basic diet:
    - o 25-30% of caloric intake as high quality protein.
    - o 40-50% of caloric intake as dietary fat (most will be associated with the protein food sources).
    - o 20-30% of calories as carbohydrate.
- Exercise:
    - o Exercises prescribed by physical therapist
    - o Exercises recommended by trainer
    - o Aerobic exercise 5 days per week; resistance exercise 2 days per week.
- EAA supplements (high leucine content):
    - o 15 grams twice per day between meals.

BIBLIOGRAPHY

1. Baum JI, Wolfe RR. The link between dietary protein intake, skeletal muscle function and health in older adults. Healthcare [Review] Jul 2015; 3(3), 529:543; doi: 10.3390/healthcare3030529
2. Weijs P, Cynober L, DeLegge M, Kreymann G, Wernerman J, Wolfe RR. Proteins and amino acids are fundamental to optimal nutrition support in critically ill patients. Crit Care [Review] Nov 2014; 18(6):591. PMID 25565377
3. Luiking YC, Ten Have GA, Wolfe RR, Deutz NE. Arginine de novo and nitric oxide production in disease states. Am J Physiol Endocrin Metab [Review] Nov 2012; 303(10):E1177-89. PMID 23011059
4. Wolfe RR, Miller SL, Miller KB. Optimal protein intake in the elderly. Clin Nutr Oct 2008. 27:675-684. PMID: 18819733
5. Wolfe RR, Miller SL. The recommended dietary allowance of protein: a misunderstood concept. JAMA Jun 2008; 299(24):2891-2893. PMID: 18577734
6. Wolfe RR. The underappreciated role of muscle in health and disease. Am J Clin Nutr [Review] Sep 2006; 84(3):475-482.
7. Wolfe RR. Skeletal muscle protein metabolism and resistance exercise. J Nutr Jan 2006; 136:525S-528S.
8. Wolfe RR. Regulation of muscle protein by amino acids. J Nutr Oct 2002; 132(10):3219S-3224S.
9. Wolfe RR. Glutamine Metabolism: Nutritional and Clinical Significance: Session II: Physiological aspects of glutamine metabolism I. J Nutr Aug 2001; 131:2496S-2497S.

10. Wolfe RR, Ferrando A, Sheffield-Moore M, Urban R. Testosterone and muscle protein metabolism. Mayo Clin Proc Jan 2000; 75:S55-S60.
11. Wolfe RR, Volpi E. Insulin and protein metabolism. Handbook of Physiology, Section 7: The Endocrine System, Volume II: The Endocrine Pancreas and Regulation of Metabolism, Oxford University Press 2001; pp 735-757.
12. Wolfe RR, Miller SL. Amino acid availability controls muscle protein metabolism. Diab Nutr Metab 1999; (5)12: 322-328.
13. Wolfe RR, Jahoor F, Hartl WH. Protein and amino acid metabolism after injury. Diabetes/Metabolism Reviews 1989; 5:149-164.
14. Wolfe RR. Does exercise stimulate protein breakdown in humans? Isotopic approaches to the problem. Med Sci Sports & Exerc 1987; 19:S172-S178.
15. Kim IY, Williams RH, Schutzler SE, Lasley CJ, Bodenner DL, Wolfe RR, Coker RH. Acute lysine supplementation does not improve hepatic or peripheral insulin sensitivity in older, overweight individuals. Nutr Metab (Lond) Oct 2014; 11(1):49. PMID:25324894
16. Witard OC, Cocke TL, Ferrando AA, Wolfe RR, Tipton KD. Increased net muscle protein balance in response to simultaneous and separate ingestion of carbohydrate and essential amino acids following resistance exercise. Appl Physiol Nutr Metab Mar 2014; 39(3):329-339. PMID:24552374
17. Engelen MPKJ, Com G, Wolfe RR, Deutz NE. Dietary essential amino acids are highly anabolic in pediatric patients with cystic fibrosis. J Cyst Fibros Sep 2013; 12(5):445-53. PMID 23357545
18. Ferrando AA, Bamman MM, Schutzler SE, Spencer HJ, Evans RP, Wolfe RR, Increased nitrogen intake following hip arthroplasty expedites muscle strength recovery. J Aging: Research Clin Practice 2013; 2(4): 369.
19. Coker RH, Miller S, Schutzler S, Deutz N, Wolfe RR. Whey protein and essential amino acids promote the reduction of adipose tissue and increased muscle protein

synthesis during caloric restriction-induced weight loss in elderly, obese individuals. Nutr J Dec 2012; 11(11):105. PMID 23231757

20. Ferrando AA, Paddon-Jones D, Hays NP, Kortebein P, Ronsen O, Williams RH, McComb A, Symons TB, Wolfe RR, Evans W. EAA supplementation to increase nitrogen intake improves muscle function during bed rest in the elderly. Clin Nutr Feb 2010; 29:18-23.

21. Katsanos CS, Aarsland A, Cree MG, Wolfe RR. Muscle protein synthesis and balance responsiveness to essential amino acids ingestion in the presence of elevated plasma free fatty acid concentrations. J Clin Endocrinol Metab Aug 2009; 94(8):2984-90. PMCID: PMC2730875

22. Børsheim E, Bui QU, Tissier S, Cree MG, Ronsen O, Morio B, Ferrando AA, Kobayashi H, Newcomer BR, Wolfe RR. Amino acid supplementation decreases plasma and liver triglycerides in elderly. Nutrition Mar 2009; 25(3):281-288. PMCID: PMC2696073

23. Zhang X-J, Chinkes DL, Wolfe RR. The anabolic effect of arginine on proteins in skin wound and muscle is independent of nitric oxide production. Clin Nutr Aug 2008; 27:649-656.

24. Borsheim E, Bui QU, Tissier S, Kobayashi H, Ferrando AA, Wolfe RR. Effect of amino acid supplementation on muscle mass, strength and physical function in elderly. Clin Nutr Apr 2008; 27(2):189-195. PMCID: PMC2430042

25. Fitts RH, Ramatowski JG, Peters JR, Paddon-Jones D, Wolfe RR, Ferrando AA. The deleterious effects of bed rest on human skeletal muscle fibers are exacerbated by hypercortisolemia and ameliorated by dietary supplementation. Am J Physiol Cell Physiol Jul 2007; 293:C313-320.

26. Killewich LA, Tuvdendorj D, Bahadorani J, GHunter GC, Wolfe RR. Amino acids stimulate leg muscle protein synthesis in peripheral arterial disease. J Vasc Surg Mar 2007; 45:554-559; discussion 559-560.

27. Katsansos CS, Kobayashi H, Sheffield-Moore M, Aarsland A, Wolfe RR. A high proportion of leucine is required for

optimal stimulation of the rate of muscle protein synthesis by essential amino acids in the elderly. Am J Physiol Endocriol Metab Aug 2006; 291:E381-E387.

28. Raj D, Welbourne T, Dominic EA, Waters D, Wolfe RR, Ferrando A. Glutamine kinetics and protein turnover in end-stage renal disease. Am J Physiol Endocrinol Metab Jul 2005; 288:E37-E46.

29. Paddon-Jones D, Sheffield-Moore M, Aarsland A, Wolfe RR, Ferrando AA. Exogenous amino acids stimulate human muscle anabolism without interfering with the response to mixed meal ingestion. Am J Physiol Apr 2005; 288(4):E761-767.

30. Paddon-Jones D, Sheffield-Moore M, Urban RJ, Aarsland A, Wolfe RR, Ferrando AA. The catabolic effects of prolonged inactivity and acute hypercortisolemia are offset by dietary supplementation. J Clin Endocrinol Metab Mar 2005; 90(3):1453-1459.

31. Paddon-Jones D, Sheffield-Moore M, Urban RJ, Sanford AP, Aarsland A, Wolfe RR, Ferrando A. Essential amino acid and carbohydrate supplementation ameliorates muscle protein loss during 28 days bedrest. J Clin Endocrinol Metabo Sep 2004; 89:4351-4358.

32. Miller SL, Chinkes DL, MacLean DA, Gore D, Wolfe RR. In vivo muscle amino acid transport involves two distinct processes. Am J Physiol Jul 2004; 287:E136-E141.

33. Paddon-Jones D, Sheffield-Moore M, Zhang X-J, Volpi E, Wolf SE, Aarsland A, Ferrando AA, Wolfe RR. Amino acid ingestion improves muscle protein synthesis in the young and elderly. Am J Physiol Mar 2004; 286:E321-E328.

34. Volpi E, Kobayashi H, Sheffield-Moore M, Mittendorfer B, Wolfe RR. Essential amino acids are primarily responsible for the amino acid stimulation of muscle protein anabolism in healthy elderly adults. Am J Clin Nutr Aug 2003; 78:250-258.

35. Tipton KD, Rasmussen B, Miller SL, Wolf SE, Owens-Stovall SK, Petrini BE, Wolfe RR. Timing of amino acid-carbohydrate ingestion alters anabolic response of muscle

to resistance exercise. Am J Physiol Aug 2001; 281:E197-E206.

36. Mittendorfer B, Volpi E, Wolfe RR. Whole-body and skeletal muscle glutamine metabolism in healthy subjects. Am J Physiol Feb 2001; 280:E323-E333.

37. Rasmussen B, Tipton KD, Miller SL, Wolf SE, Wolfe RR. An oral essential amino acid - carbohydrate supplement enhances muscle protein anabolism after resistance exercise. J Appl Physiol Feb 2000; 88(2): 386-39.

38. Volpi E, Mittendorfer B, Wolf SE, Wolfe RR. Oral amino acids stimulate muscle protein anabolism in elderly despite higher first-pass splanchnic extraction. Am J Physiology 1999; 277:E513-E520.

39. Biolo G, Williams BD, Fleming RYD, Wolfe RR. Insulin action on muscle protein kinetics and amino acid transport during recovery after resistance exercise. Diabetes 1999; 48:949-957.acids are not necessary to stimulate net muscle protein synthesis in healthy volunteers. J Nutr Biochem 1999; 10:89-95.

40. Tipton, KD, Ferrando AA, Phillips SM, Doyle D, Jr, Wolfe RR. Post exercise net protein synthesis in human muscle from orally administered amino acids. Am J Physiol 276(Endocrinol Metab 39), E628-E634, 1999.

41. Phillips SM, Tipton KD, Ferrando AA, Wolfe RR. Resistance training reduces the acute exercise-induced increase in muscle protein turnover. Am J Physiol 276 (Endocrinol Metab 39):E118-E124, 1999.

42. Williams BD, Chinkes DL, Wolfe RR. Alanine and glutamine kinetics at rest and during exercise in humans. Med Sci Sports Exerc 1998; 30(7):1053-1058.

43. Volpi E, Ferrando AA, Yeckel CW, Tipton KD, Wolfe RR. Exogenous amino acids stimulate net muscle protein synthesis in the elderly. J Clin Invest 1998; 101(9):2000-2007.

44. Biolo G, Tipton KD, Klein S, Wolfe RR. An abundant supply of amino acids enhances the metabolic effect of exercise on muscle protein. Am J Physiol 273 (Endocrinol Metab 36): E122-E129, 1997

45. Phillips SM, Tipton KD, Aarsland A, Wolf SE, Wolfe RR. Mixed muscle protein synthesis and breakdown after resistance exercise in humans. Am J Physiol 273 (Endocrinol Metab 36): E99-E107, 1997.

46. Tipton KD, Ferrando AA, Williams BD, Wolfe RR. Muscle protein metabolism in female swimmers after a combination of resistance and endurance exercise. J Appl Physiol 1996; 81:2034-2038.

47. Williams BD, Wolfe RR, Bracy DP, Wasserman DH. Gut proteolysis contributes essential amino acids during exercise. Am. J. Physiol. 270 (Endocrino. Metab. 33):E85-E90, 1996.

48. Biolo G, Zhang X-J, Wolfe RR. Role of membrane transport in inter organ amino acid flow between muscle and small intestine. Metabolism 1995; 44(6):719-724.

49. Biolo G, Wolfe RR. Relationship between plasma amino acid kinetics and tissue protein synthesis and breakdown. Proc. IFAC Symp on Modeling and Control in Biological Systems, ed. B. W. Patterson. Madison:Omnipress, 1994; pp. 358-359.

50. Biolo G, Maggi SP, Williams BD, Tipton K, Wolfe RR. Increased rates of muscle protein turnover and amino acid transport after resistance exercise in humans. Am J Physiol 268 (Endocrinol. Metab. 31):E514-E520, 1995

51. Biolo G, Fleming RYD, Wolfe RR. Physiologic hyperinsulinemia stimulates protein synthesis and enhances transport of selected amino acids in human skeletal muscle. J Clin Invest 1995; 95:811-819.

52. Biolo G, Gastaldeli A, Zhang X-J, Wolfe RR. Protein synthesis and breakdown in skin and muscle: a leg model of amino acid kinetics. Am. J. Physiol. 267(Endocrinol. Metab. 30):E467-E474, 1994.

53. Kobayashi H, Borsheim E, Traber DL, Badalamenti J, Anthony TG, Kimball SR, Jefferson LS, Wolfe RR. Reduced amino acid availability inhibits muscle protein synthesis by a mechanism involving initiation factor eIF2B. Am J Physiol Mar 2003; 84:E488-E498.

54. Romijn, JA, Coyle EF, Sidossis EF, Gastaldelli A, Horowitz JF, Endert E, Wolfe RR. Regulation of

endogenous fat and carbohydrate metabolism in relation to exercise intensity and duration. Am. J. Physiol. 265(Endocrinol. Metab. 28):E380-E391, 1993

55. Carraro F, Hartl WH, Stuart CA, Layman DK, Jahoor F, Wolfe RR. Whole body and plasma protein synthesis in exercise and recovery in human subjects. Am J Physiol 1990; 258:E821-E831.

56. Stein TP, Hoyt RW, Toole MO, Leskiw MJ, Schutler MD, Wolfe RR, Hiller WD. Protein and energy metabolism during prolonged exercise in trained athletes. Int J Sports Med 1989; 10:311-316.

57. Wolfe RR, Jahoor F, Shaw JH. Effect of alanine infusion on glucose and urea production in man. J Parent Enteral Nutr 1987; 11:109-111.

58. Shaw JH, Klein S, Wolfe RR. Assessment of alanine, urea, and glucose interrelationships in normal subjects and in patients with sepsis with stable isotopic tracers. Surgery 1985; 97:557-568.

59. Wolfe RR, Wolfe MH, Nadel ER, Shaw JH. Isotopic determination of amino acid-urea interactions in exercise in humans. J Appl Physiol 1984; 56:221-229.

60. Paddon-Jones D, Sheffield-Moore M, Zhang X-J, Katsanos CS, Wolfe RR. Differential stimulation of muscle protein synthesis in elderly humans following isocaloric ingestion of amino acids or whey protein. Exp Gerontol 2006; 41:215-219.

61. Dillon EL, Sheffield-Moere M, Paddon-Jones D, Gilkison X, Sanford AP, Casperson SL, Jiang J, Chinkes DL, Urban, RJ. Amino acid supplementation increases lean body mass, basal muscle protein synthesis, and insulin-like growth factor 1 expression in older women. J Clin Endo. Metab 2009; 94: 1630-7.

62. Bukhari SS, Phillips BE, Wilkinson DJ, Limb MC, Rankin D, Mitchell WK, Kobayashi H, Greenhaff P, Smith K, Atherton PJ. Intake of low-dose leucine-rich essential amino acids stimulates muscle anabolism equivalently to bolus whey protein in older women at rest and after exercise. Am J Physiol Endo and Metab 2015; 308: E1056-65.

63. Patterson BW, Nguyen T, Pierre E, Herndon DN, Wolfe RR. Urea and protein metabolism in burned children: effect of dietary protein intake. Metabolism 1997; 46, 5:573-578.

64. Coker RH, Deutz NE, Schutzler S, Beggs M, Miller S, Wolfe RR, Wei J. Nutritional supplementation with essential amino acids and phytosterols may reduce risk of metabolic syndrome and cardiovascular disease in overweight individuals with mild hyperlipidemia. J Endocrinol Diabetes Obes 3(2): pii: 1069, Epub 2015 Apr 15. PMID:2672631

65. Tipton KD, Gurkin BE, Matin S, Wolfe, RR.Non-essential acids are not necessary to stimulate net muscle protein synthesis in healthy volunteers. J Nutr Biochem 1999; 10:89-95.

66. Kim JE, O'Connor LE, Sands, LP, Slebodnik MB, Campbell WW. Effect of dietary protein intake on body composition changes after weight loss in older (over 50 years of age) adults: a systematic review and meta-analysis. Nutrition Reviews 2016;74:210-224.

67. Kim IY, Park S, Chou TH, Trombold RS, Coyle EF. Prolonged sitting negatively affects the post-prandial plasma-triglyceride lowering effect of acute exercise. Am J Physiol 2016;E891-E8998.

68. The Brain: Understanding Neurobiology. https://science.education.nih.gov.

69. Kohrt WM, Holloszy JO. Loss of skeletal muscle mass with aging: effect on glucose tolerance. J Gerontol A Biol Sci Med Sci 1995; Spec No:68-72.

GLOSSARY

Amino acid - a simple organic compound containing both a carboxyl (-COOH) and an amino (-NH2) group. There are 20 amino acids important in human nutrition and metabolism.

Adenosine triphosphate (ATP) - nucleotide that is the primary source of energy in all living cells because of its function in donating a phosphate group during biochemical activities.

Anabolism - the net gain of muscle protein (protein synthesis is greater than protein breakdown).

Anabolic state - the condition in which muscle mass is increasing (stimulation of anabolism).

Anabolic resistance - when the normal anabolic effect of dietary protein is diminished or lost. This is the case in aging and the stress response.

BCAAs - branched chain amino acids leucine, isoleucine, and valine.

Calorie - unit used in relation to energy production by the body and dietary energy consumption. Technically the term is Kilocalorie, and thus the standard abbreviation of kcal.

Catabolism - net loss of muscle protein.

Catabolic state – a condition in which muscle is being broken down (acceleration of catabolism).

Deoxyribonucleic acid (DNA) - DNA is the hereditary material in humans and almost all other organisms. Every cell in a person's body has the same DNA. Most DNA is located in the cell nucleus (where it is called nuclear DNA), but a small amount of DNA can also be found in the mitochondria (where it is called mitochondrial DNA or mtDNA).

Essential amino acid (EAA) - an essential amino acid or indispensable amino acid is an amino acid that cannot be synthesized (from scratch) in the body, and thus must be supplied by the diet.

Enzyme - a specialized protein that makes a metabolic reaction go faster in the body.

Metabolism - a general term referring to the biochemical degradation of molecules in the body.

Metabolite - a substance produced in a metabolic reaction.

Mitochondria - structures located inside the cell. Mitochondria are the place in the cell where energy is produced. Not only are nutrients converted into energy in mitochondria but other specialized tasks are performed in mitochondria as well.

Muscle Protein Synthesis - protein synthesis is the process by which amino acids are linearly attached into a chain of prescribed length and composition. Muscle protein synthesis refers to the building of muscle protein by combining amino acids to form skeletal muscle.

Muscle Protein Breakdown - the breakdown of skeletal muscle proteins into the component amino acids. Muscle protein breakdown occurs continuously and is accelerated in states of inadequate caloric intake or catabolic disease. Breakdown occurs to provide the organism with amino acids essential for gluconeogenesis, new protein synthesis and energy production.

mTOR - "mammalian target of rapamycin" (mTOR) is an intracellular signaling molecule that regulates a variety of functions related to cell growth.

Non-essential amino acid (NEAA) - an amino acid that can be made by humans and so is not essential to the human diet.

Precursor - a substance from which another is formed, especially by metabolic reaction. For example, amino acids are precursors for protein synthesis.

Substrate – molecule on which an enzyme acts in a metabolic reaction. While *substrate* can refer to any molecule involved in a metabolic reaction, in this book *substrate* refers to molecules that can be metabolized to produce ATP, and thus energy. Carbohydrates and fats are the primary energy substrates.

APPENDIX

The Amino Acids

Essential Amino Acids (EAAs)

EAAs must be consumed as part of the diet, because the body either cannot make them at all or enough to meet demand. Animal-based proteins such as meat, chicken, dairy and fish are excellent sources of EAAs.

Leucine. Leucine is one of three branched-chain amino acids (BCAA). The term *branched chain* refers to the chemical structure. Isoleucine and valine are the other two BCAAs. Leucine is the best known of the BCAAs. Leucine is the most abundant EAA in muscle. In addition, leucine acts as a signal to activate various functions of the cells, including starting the process of protein synthesis. Leucine can activate the process of protein synthesis by activating a group of intracellular compounds collectively known as *initiation factors*. The key initiation factor activated by leucine is called mTOR. Activation of mTOR acts as a sensor in the cell. When the leucine concentration in the cell increases after consumption of leucine, mTOR is activated. Activation of mTOR can increase the amount of muscle protein that is produced, provided there are enough of the other EAAs available to make complete proteins. When leucine concentrations are low, it signals mTOR that there is not enough dietary protein present to synthesize new skeletal muscle protein and it is deactivated. As the leucine concentration increases, it signals to mTOR that there is sufficient dietary protein to synthesize new skeletal muscle protein and mTOR is activated. While mTOR activation is not always linked with increased protein synthesis, it is an anabolic signal when all the necessary components are present. Because of the regulatory role leucine plays in controlling metabolism above and beyond its importance as a precursor for protein synthesis, leucine is often referred to as a *nutraceutical*. Leucine serves other functions as well. Leucine contributes to the regulation of blood-sugar levels; growth and repair of muscle and bone tissue; growth hormone production; and wound healing. Leucine also prevents breakdown of muscle proteins after trauma or severe stress. Leucine can increase the number of mitochondria in muscle. Mitochondria are the organelles in muscle where the ATP is generated to fuel muscle contraction during exercise.

Isoleucine. Isoleucine is one of the other BCAAs. Isoleucine contains the exact same number of carbon, oxygen, nitrogen, and hydrogen atoms as leucine. The two amino acids are distinguished only by the conformation of the molecules. Despite the chemical similarities between leucine and isoleucine, there are clear differences between the function of the two molecules. Unlike leucine, isoleucine doesn't seem to play a role in regulating protein synthesis or other metabolic reactions. The principal role of isoleucine is as a component of protein, particularly muscle protein. Isoleucine also contributes to other diverse physiological functions, such as assisting in wound healing and hemoglobin synthesis.

Valine. Valine is the third BCAA. Like the other BCAAs and EAAs, valine promotes muscle growth and tissue repair. Although not a physiological function, it is interesting that valine is a precursor in the penicillin biosynthetic pathway. Valine helps to determine the three-dimensional structure of proteins. The claims that valine helps to maintain mental vigor, muscle coordination, and emotional calm are common, but I could find little evidence to support these claims. Valine is believed to play a part in the central nervous system and cognitive functioning because it influences the transport of molecules into the brain. Valine, like alanine, can also remove excess nitrogen from the liver and transport it to other areas of the body where needed.

BCAAs. Leucine, isoleucine and valine have different roles in some respects, but it is worthwhile to consider some of the commonalities, as those are the basis for the large demand for nutritional supplements of BCAAs. All three BCAAs are abundant in body proteins, particularly skeletal muscle. High quality dietary proteins are defined in part by the amount of BCAAS contained in the protein. The BCAAs are metabolized in the muscle, meaning that they can be oxidized and used as a fuel source during prolonged endurance exercise. They are often promoted to athletes for this reason. The BCAAs are also promoted as dietary

286

supplements because they stimulate muscle protein synthesis, but this can only happen if all of the other EAAs are consumed at the same time. All three BCAAs influence brain function by modifying large, neutral amino acid (LNAA) transport into the brain. Transport is shared by different groups of amino acids and is competitive. Consequently, when plasma BCAA concentrations rise, for example after consumption of a dietary supplement of BCAAs, brain BCAA concentrations rises, and the concentration of tryptophan declines. These changes inhibit the production of the neurotransmitter serotonin.

Lysine. As in the case of all the EAAs, lysine is required for growth and tissue repair. Lysine is an important component of muscle protein. You need to consume more lysine than you might think from the recommended dietary intake. This is because some dietary lysine may be altered during digestion so that the body cannot use it. Also once lysine is in the blood, it is transported into muscle very sluggishly. Therefore, you need to consume more lysine to achieve the optimal balance of EAAs inside the muscle cells than you would think from the composition of muscle protein. In addition to its important role as a precursor for protein synthesis, lysine plays a particularly important role in the immune system. It is involved in the development of antibodies and has important antiviral properties. As a nutritional supplement, lysine seems to be active against herpes simplex viruses (HSV). The mechanism underlying this effect is based on the need for the virus to obtain arginine. Lysine competes with arginine for absorption and entry into cells and thereby inhibits HSV growth. A lysine deficiency is characterized by broken skin, fragile nails and in extreme cases loss of hair. There is also evidence that lysine increases the effectiveness of arginine in promoting human growth hormone (HGH) release. While lysine is supplied by many animal proteins (red meats, fish, and dairy products), it is typically the limiting amino acid in plant proteins. Vegetarians and especially vegans must be diligent in choosing proteins or opt for supplements to ensure adequate lysine intake.

Methionine. Methionine is a sulfur-containing amino acid that is important in many body functions. Methionine occupies a

287

unique position among the EAAs regarding its role in protein synthesis. The process of protein synthesis involves a sequential stringing together of the component amino acids in a precise order dictated by the messenger RNA (mRNA) in the cell. Methionine is always the first amino acid transcribed from the mRNA. Consequently, without adequate methionine availability, the synthesis of protein never gets started. Despite this crucial role in protein synthesis, methionine is not often the limiting amino acid in protein synthesis. In addition to its role in protein synthesis, methionine is particularly essential for many structural and metabolic functions. This is because of the sulfur side group. The cartilage in the joints requires sulfur for its production. Studies have shown that the cartilage from healthy people contains approximately three times more sulfur than in arthritis patients. Sulfur cannot be taken in tablet form or as a dietary supplement but methionine is a safe dietary approach to take in sulfur. Owing to its capacity to form sulfurous chains which in turn connect with each other, methionine is able to strengthen the structure of hair and nails. Beyond stimulating the formation of cartilage tissue, methionine also has anti-inflammatory and analgesic properties. Sulfur provided by methionine protects cells from pollutants and slows cell aging, in part by its involvement in many detoxifying processes. It is essential for the absorption and bio-availability of selenium and zinc. Methionine aids in detoxification and excretion of chemicals such as lead and mercury. In balance with the other sulfur-containing amino acid cysteine, methionine is important for liver health by minimizing the accumulation of fat in the liver.

Threonine. Threonine is an important component of many proteins, such as tooth enamel, collagen, and elastin. Threonine is used to create glycine and serine, two amino acids that are directly involved in the production of collagen, elastin, and muscle tissue. Threonine helps keep connective tissues and muscles throughout the body strong and elastic. It also helps build strong bones and tooth enamel, and may speed wound healing or recovery from injury. Threonine plays an important role in fat metabolism and prevents fat accumulation in the liver. It combines with the amino acids aspartic acid and methionine to help the liver with the metabolism of fats and fatty acids. Without enough threonine in

288

the body, fats build up in the liver, predisposing the liver to scarring and potential liver failure. Supplements are proposed to be useful for intestinal disorders and indigestion, and the presumed mechanism relates to enhanced digestion, but this function is not well documented. Threonine can act to increase glycine levels in the central nervous system even better than administering glycine, since glycine itself cannot cross into the central nervous system.

Phenylalanine. Phenylalanine is important in the structure and function of many proteins and enzymes. It is a precursor of another amino acid, tyrosine. Tyrosine is converted into a number of brain chemicals including dopamine, epinephrine, norepinephrine, and thyroid hormones. Norepinephrine, epinephrine and dopamine affect mood, focus, and other facets of brain function so different forms of phenylalanine have been proposed to treat mood disorders, stress, anxiety and pain. Phenylalanine is a component of the artificial sweetener Aspartame (aspartate is the other amino acid component). A small percentage of people lack the enzyme to metabolize phenylalanine and must restrict the amount they consume to avoid high circulating levels of phenylalanine.

Tryptophan. Tryptophan is necessary for normal growth in infants and for maintaining a balance between protein synthesis and breakdown in adults. Tryptophan is widely recognized as a precursor of the neurotransmitter serotonin, hence its use as an antidepressant and sleep aid. Tryptophan is converted to 5-hydroxy-tryptophan (5-HTP) which is, in turn, converted to serotonin, a neurotransmitter essential in regulating appetite, sleep, mood, and pain. Tryptophan deficiency can cause depression. A tryptophan deficiency is not very common, as the requirement is low relative to other EAAs, but certain meal substitute formulations used for weight loss programs were low in tryptophan. As a result, participants in these programs got depressed even though they were losing weight. Tryptophan can also be a precursor to vitamin B3 (niacin) although it is not used very efficiently in this manner.

Histidine. Histidine may be considered a semi-essential amino acid because children require dietary sources while adults can produce some histidine but not enough to meet requirements. However, histidine is classified as an EAA because a diet deficient in histidine will limit growth and development in children, and create a problem in adults if rates of histidine synthesis do not match the rates of breakdown. Histidine has many vital functions within the body. It is involved in the synthesis of hemoglobin, tissue repair and the strengthening of the immune system among other functions. In the central nervous system, it is important for the maintenance of myelin sheaths that protect nerve cells. Histidine is also metabolized to the neurotransmitter histamine. Histamine plays many roles in immunity and gastric function via production of secretions. It is also important for sexual functions due to its influence on blood flow. This is why you don't want to take an anti-histamine before a romantic interlude.

Semi-essential amino acids are normally not required in the diet because the body can produce them at an adequate rate. In some circumstances, often related to stressors such as disease or exercise training, the body cannot produce an adequate amount to meet all demands.

Arginine. Arginine is considered semi-essential in that it is required in infants and children. Adults can synthesize arginine, but in stressful condition such as serious illness or injury, the body may not be able to meet demands; thus, dietary sources are required. The problem is that a great deal of arginine absorbed from the intestine after consumption is directly taken up by the liver, and therefore arginine availability is not increased in the parts of the body in which it is needed. For that reason, the amino acid citrulline may be provided to increase arginine availability. Citrulline is an unusual amino acid in that it is produced in the body in the production of urea, but it is not a component of body protein. Furthermore, citrulline is not contained in almost any dietary proteins (watermelon protein surprisingly is a source of dietary citrulline). Consequently, the production of arginine may become limited by the availability of its precursor citrulline. Providing citrulline as a dietary supplement will increase arginine in the blood much more than consumption of arginine itself, since citrulline is not cleared by the liver, but rather is taken up by the kidney, where it is converted to arginine. Arginine is a precursor for nitric oxide, which is a vasodilator that relaxes blood vessels and is therefore useful in treating angina and circulatory diseases. Arginine is the component of protein that can help to lower blood pressure by stimulating nitric oxide production. Arginine also helps with erectile function in men, again related to its effect on blood flow. In addition, nitric oxide from arginine increases the proportion of blood flow that goes to the muscle, thereby increasing the delivery of nutrients and clearing of waste products. Arginine is an important intermediate in detoxification of nitrogenous wastes by playing a central role in conversion of these potentially-toxic compounds to (non-toxic) urea and eventual excretion in the urine.

Glutamine. Glutamine is synthesized from glutamic acid and ammonia. It is normally present in relatively high concentrations throughout the body and is involved in many metabolic processes. It is the principal carrier of nitrogen in the body and is an important energy source for many cells. Glutamine regulates ammonia by carrying it as a side chain and using it in the formation of urea for eventual excretion by the kidneys. Glutamine can serve as a substrate for the production of both excitatory and inhibitory neurotransmitters (glutamate and GABA) and is also an important source of energy for the nervous system. Cells of the small intestine and mucosa rely on glutamine as a fuel source and supplements may help to manage symptoms of leaky gut. As in the case of arginine, dietary glutamine may become an essential amino acid during certain stressful states. Glutamine is normally the most abundant free amino acid in the muscle, and depletion of muscle glutamine is an indicator of the "overtraining syndrome". Muscle glutamine depletion is also the hallmark of muscle wasting in critical illness. Unfortunately, consumption of dietary glutamine may not readily reverse depletion of the glutamine in the muscle, since the depletion arises because of a metabolic defect that tends to keep glutamine out of the muscle even when supplied via the diet.

Tyrosine. Tyrosine is synthesized in vivo from phenylalanine. It is considered a non-essential amino acid, but in the rare circumstance in which the chemical pathway from phenylalanine to tyrosine is not functional then tyrosine must be consumed in the diet. Also, if phenylalanine requirements are not met by the diet, tyrosine availability is limited and may be required from food sources. In addition to its role in protein synthesis, tyrosine is involved in the production of thyroid hormones and neurotransmitters such as dopamine, norepinephrine and epinephrine. These neurotransmitters play a vital role in the nervous system and in the management of stress and depression. Tyrosine is used as a safe therapy for a variety of clinical conditions including hypertension, depression, and chronic pain.

These functions are accomplished by facilitating the synthesis of peptides and enkephalins that act as the body's natural pain relievers. Tyrosine can also be used as an add-on in the treatment of Parkinson's disease. L-dopa, which is used in the treatment of Parkinson's, is the intermediary product of tyrosine before dopamine.

Non-Essential Amino Acids (NEAAs)

NEAAs are produced at a rate sufficient to meet the bodies demand and are therefore not required in the diet. Nonetheless, consumption of some NEAAs in the diet aids in the production of new protein. Since almost all dietary proteins contain more NEAAs than EAAs, we normally get the majority of NEAAs in our body by eating protein.

Alanine. Alanine is the smallest amino acid in humans and is readily synthesised in the body. Alanine plays a unique role in the transfer of nitrogen from muscles and peripheral tissues to the liver. In the muscle, a compound called pyruvate combines with nitrogen to form the amino acid alanine. Circulating alanine is then taken up by the liver where the nitrogen is removed and used to form other NEAAs or is directed to urea production. The pyruvate then can be oxidized for energy or converted to glucose to be used throughout the body. This cycle is referred to as the glucose-alanine cycle. Alanine, therefore, is an important source of energy for muscles and the central nervous system. It is also second only to glutamine in the amount circulating in the blood. Alanine helps to produce lymphocytes which are cells in lymph fluid and the bloodstream and are involved in immune function.

Asparagine. Asparagine is biosynthesized from aspartic acid and ammonia. Asparagine is readily converted back to aspartic acid. Asparagine can act as a neurotransmitter and, along with aspartate, maintains balance in the central nervous system. Asparagine is a component of many proteins including glycoproteins. Glycoproteins are specialized structures that provide many functions: they give structural support to cells, help to form connective tissues and facilitate digestion by producing secretions and mucous in the gastrointestinal tract.

Aspartic Acid. Aspartic acid works in the brain, alongside asparagine, as an excitatory neurotransmitter. It plays an important role in the synthesis of other amino acids and in metabolic reactions involved in energy production (the citric acid cycle) and the production of urea. Aspartic acid is a part of the chemical structure of the active part of many enzymes. Enzymes are specialized proteins that play a role in enabling chemical reactions to occur in the body. Many other amino acids are synthesized from aspartic acid.

Cysteine. Cysteine, like methionine, is distinctive in that it contains sulfur. It is important for protein synthesis, detoxification, and other diverse functions. It is abundant in the protein beta-keratin, the main protein in nails, skin, and hair, Cysteine is also important in collagen production. Collagen protein is a major component of the skin and connective tissue, and helps to maintain the elasticity and texture of skin. For this reason, cysteine supplements are sometimes marketed as anti-aging products that claim to stimulate the formation of collagen and improve skin elasticity. Cysteine supplementation may also help speed the healing of burns and wounds, and improve joint flexibility in those with rheumatoid arthritis. Cysteine is required in the production of taurine. Taurine is a sulfur-containing compound that is a constituent of bile. Taurine also plays a role as an antioxidant, and is essential for cardiovascular and skeletal muscle function. One of the most important roles of cysteine is that it is a component of the antioxidant glutathione. Glutathione is an all-important anti-oxidant used throughout the body to neutralize free radicals and diminish oxidative stress. It is particularly important in detoxification processes in the liver. One form of cysteine, n-acetyl-L-cysteine (NAC) is typically given as a supplement or medication to promote the production of glutathione. After absorption, NAC is converted to cysteine and then to glutathione. NAC in pharmacological doses is used to treat acetaminophen poisoning, angina, and respiratory conditions.

Glutamic Acid. Glutamic acid or glutamate is the most common excitatory neurotransmitter in the central nervous system. It serves as an energy source for brain cells. Glutamate is a close cousin of glutamine (see above), in that they share the same chemical structure except that glutamine has one additional N group. Glutamate and glutamine are readily interconverted. In the brain, glutamate can regulate ammonia levels by taking up nitrogen in its conversion to glutamine, another amino acid that functions as a neurotransmitter. Glutamate serves the same function in the periphery, taking up ammonia and then carrying it via the blood back to the liver for ultimate conversion to urea which is then excreted. Glutamic acid is also important in the synthesis of gamma-aminobutyric acid (GABA). An inhibitory neurotransmitter, GABA has the opposite effect of glutamic acid and helps to decrease activity within the central nervous system.

Glycine. Glycine is a *glucogenic* amino acid meaning it is a precursor for the production of glucose by the liver. We need to have a constant level of glucose in the blood, as this is the energy source of the brain and even a transient dip in glucose concentration can result in a drop in brain function. Since we eat meals intermittently, the liver must produce glucose in the intervals between meals to avoid a drop in plasma glucose concentration. Amino acids are crucial in this process. Glycine is one of several "glucogenic" amino acids. Structurally, glycine is a very simple amino acid since its side group is a single hydrogen. Glycine is the second most common amino acid in human proteins. For example, approximately one third of collagen is comprised of glycine. Collagen is the predominant protein required to keep the connective tissue and skin flexible and firm. In addition to its role as a major component of most proteins, glycine helps in the breakdown of ingested fats by regulating the secretion of bile acids from the gall bladder into the small intestine. Glycine accomplishes several functions as a neurotransmitter in the CNS. It is also an inhibitory neurotransmitter that participates in the processing of motor and sensory information that permits movement, vision, and hearing.

Proline. Proline is synthesized from glutamic acid and other amino acids. Proline is a constituent of many proteins. Almost one-third of the amino acids in collagen are proline. Proline production increases during times of soft-tissue trauma, injury and wound healing, such as muscle or tendon recovery, severe burns and after surgery. Proline is also promoted for arteriosclerosis prevention and blood pressure maintenance. Arteriosclerosis occurs when the blood vessels, or arteries, that carry oxygen and

296

nutrients from the heart to the rest of your body become thick and stiff from the build-up of fat on artery walls. This prevents the artery from expanding and contracting when your heart beats and can restrict blood flow to your organs and tissues. Proline enables the walls to release fat build-up into the bloodstream, decreasing the size of the blockages to the heart and surrounding vessels. Proline, therefore, decreases the pressure built up by these blockages, decreasing blood pressure and the risk of heart disease.

Serine. Serine is synthesized from glycine or threonine and is present and functionally important in many proteins. Serine helps produce immunoglobulins and antibodies for a strong immune system, and also aids in the absorption of creatine. Creatine is a substance made from amino acids that helps build and maintain all the muscles in the body, including the heart. Serine is needed for the metabolism of fats and fatty acids. Serine is part of the structure of trypsin and chymotrypsin, two major digestive enzymes needed to breakdown protein from foods that we eat. Cell membranes rely on serine since it forms the phospholipids needed to encase cells throughout the body. Serine is important for both physical and mental functioning but it is especially important for proper functioning of the brain and central nervous system.

Non-Dietary Amino Acids in the Body

The above amino acids are all found in body protein, and we refer to them as dietary amino acids. This terminology is to distinguish them from other amino acids in the body that have important metabolic roles that are not incorporated into body proteins. A number of amino acids fall into this category. None of the non-dietary amino acids are considered essential and there are no dietary guidelines recommending levels of intake. Nonetheless, certain non-dietary amino acids are frequent components of nutritional supplements. I will focus on three of these non-dietary amino acids.

Carnitine. Carnitine is produced in the body from the amino acids lysine and methionine. Carnitine is necessary for the metabolism of fatty acids for energy. Fatty acids must be transported into organelles in cells called mitochondria, where the biochemical process of energy production occurs. Carnitine is required for the transport of fatty acids into the mitochondria.

Creatine. Creatine helps to provide energy to all cells in the body, but particularly muscle. Creatine phosphate is a readily available source for the production of ATP in muscle, which provides the energy for muscle contraction.

Citrulline. Citrulline is one of the three amino acids in the urea cycle, which (as the name implies), is involved in the production of urea from nitrogenous products of amino acid metabolism. The other two amino acids that are part of the urea cycle are ornithine (another non-dietary amino acid in the body) and arginine. Citrulline is formed as a consequence of the production of nitric oxide from arginine. The cyclic nature of the relationship between arginine and citrulline means that while citrulline is produced from the metabolism of arginine, citrulline in turn serves as the precursor for the production of arginine. The availability of citrulline seems to be rate limiting for the production of arginine, because consumption of citrulline increases arginine concentration in the blood. In turn, the increase in

298

arginine availability increases the production of citrulline and nitric oxide.

Made in the USA
Middletown, DE
31 August 2018